Values in Conflict
Resolving Ethical Issues in Hospital Care

Report of the Special Committee on Biomedical Ethics

American Hospital Association
840 North Lake Shore Drive
Chicago, Illinois 60611

AHA

Values in Conflict
Resolving Ethical Issues in Hospital Care
The Report of the General Council Special Committee
on Biomedical Ethics

*Values in Conflict: Resolving Ethical Issues in Hospital
Care,* Report of the Special Committee on Biomedical
Ethics, was approved by the General Council of the
American Hospital Association on April 10, 1985. It has
the status of Association guidelines, providing general
advice to hospitals on development of policies and procedures relating to biomedical ethics.

Library of Congress Cataloging in Publication Data

American Hospital Association. Special Committee on
   Biomedical Ethics.
   Values in conflict.

   Includes bibliographies and index.
   1. Medical ethics. 2. Hospital care—Moral and
ethical aspects. I. Title. [DNLM: 1. Delivery of
Health Care—standards—United States. 2. Ethics,
Medical. 3. Hospitals—standards—United States.
W 50 A5126v]
R725.5.A45 1985   362.1'1'0218   85-14213
ISBN 0-87258-433-X

January 1985

To: General Council

Subject: *Values in Conflict:*
Resolving Ethical Issues in Hospital Care
Report of the Special Committee on Biomedical Ethics

I am pleased to submit this final report of the Special
Committee on Biomedical Ethics. On behalf of the entire
committee, I want to express our appreciation for the
trust and confidence that the General Council exhibited
in establishing this committee with such an important
task. At all times, we were guided by the goal to assist
hospitals in developing policies and procedures to deal
with ethical dilemmas in modern health care. At the same
time, we recognized the immensity of this challenge, and
that our work could only be a prelude to future efforts of
the American Hospital Association.

The committee chose to confine its activities to ethical
issues directly related to providing patient services. It in-
tentionally omitted consideration of biomedical ethical
issues inherent in research, questions as to whether a
given type of service is ethical (genetic engineering,
genetic screening, artificial reproduction, etc.), and broad
challenges facing society as a whole such as ethical
distribution of the nation's health care resources. Even so,
the committee felt almost overwhelmed at the range of
critical issues confronting it. However, our task was aided
immeasurably by the assistance of a superb staff.

It is the committee's sincere hope that the report will
help hospitals to create an environment in which the
ethical challenges in patient care delivery can be met in a
compassionate and morally responsible manner that is
sensitive to the needs of patients, their families, health
care professionals, and the hospital.

Paul B. Hofmann
Chairman
Special Committee on Biomedical Ethics

92634

General Council Special Committee on Biomedical Ethics*

Paul B. Hofmann, chairman
Christine I. Mitchell, R.N., vice-chairman
Stanley S. Bergen, Jr., M.D.
Bob L. Bybee
Robert M. Cunningham, Jr.
Dorothy Danielson, R.N.
William G. Gordon
Joanne Lynn, M.D.
Kenneth A. Marshall
Rev. Richard A. McCormick, S.J.
Marcella L. O'Halloran
John A. Reinertsen
Rabbi Seymour Siegel
Mark Siegler, M.D.
Rt. Rev. William B. Spofford, Jr.

Edward W. Weimer, secretary
Michael Lesparre, assistant secretary
Gail Lovinger, assistant secretary

Richard L. Epstein, counsel to the Special Committee

* See Roster, Appendix A

Contents

Introduction: About This Report

In the past decade the ethical implications of health care treatment and delivery have raised difficult and important questions for health care institutions. The complexity and number of ethical dilemmas have grown substantially because of the increasing sophistication of medical science and technology, concern about practical limits on financial resources for health care, changes in society, and growing emphasis on the autonomy of the individual.

The American Hospital Association's continuing interest in biomedical ethical issues prompted the General Council to establish the Special Committee on Biomedical Ethics with the following charge:

- To identify the major biomedical ethical issues facing hospitals
- To formulate guidelines to assist hospitals in developing institutional policies and processes for decision making on biomedical ethical issues

Hospital Role in Biomedical Ethics

By virtue of its mission, its historical roots in charitable and religious organizations, and its fiduciary commitment to each patient and the community, the hospital is usually perceived to have a particular, if assumed, moral responsibility for health care. First, as a medical institution, the hospital has responsibility for supervision and review of patient care. The hospital must ensure that standards of quality are met and make certain that the basic processes that characterize relationships and decisions between patients and health care professionals are consistent with sound ethical principles.

Second, as a health care provider and an employer with a commitment to patient care, the hospital must develop policies and mechanisms through which questions of human values may be addressed. Third, as a center of health care delivery in the community, the hospital often must respond responsibly to social problems and dilemmas that affect the demand and need for health care services.

These roles all reinforce the need for a coherent, institutionwide approach to ethical issues that arise in patient care.

Hospital Policies Concerning Biomedical Ethics

Hospitals must develop, implement, and support institutional policies that acknowledge and address major ethical issues in providing patient care. These policies should be consistent with the institution's mission and provide the basis for resolving conflicts and questions regarding differing values. They should be sensitive to community standards regarding treatment modalities and attitudes and customs related to illness and death.

These policies also should serve as the basis for education programs to assist physicians and other health care professionals in the hospital to recognize when potentially difficult biomedical ethical issues are likely to arise. In addition, education should inform those working and volunteering in the hospital about the acceptable range of practices, attitudes, and decisions that, in effect, establish the biomedical ethical environment of the hospital. These policies should be reviewed periodically to ensure they remain relevant and appropriate.

Hospital policies and practices should respect the patient's responsibility for decision making, and should support the appropriate roles of patients, their families, and various health care professionals in decisions about care and treatment. The needs and information that other health care professionals, particularly those involved in direct care of the patient, and the patient's family may bring to the decision-making process should not be overlooked. Policies should recognize the role, knowledge, and expertise of nurses, social workers, patient representatives, chaplains, and others who may have important perspectives and expertise to offer. Policies should encourage development of a hospital environment in which appropriate members of the health care team share information and consult with each other on ethical questions affecting a patient's care. To the extent that the patient is willing to involve family members, hospital policies should support such involvement.

Hospital policies and practices should stress that the personal liberties of patients and those involved in patient care must be respected. At the same time, policies also must make it clear that the hospital setting may place legitimate limits and restrictions on those liberties, and should identify when and how those limits may be applied.

Hospital policies should emphasize that, whenever possible, dilemmas and conflicts should be resolved at the level closest to the patient, at the lowest cost, and ordinarily without resort to the courts. This is usually the best way to assure that decisions comply with the patient's own values and needs. Bringing a patient care treatment decision into the courts restricts the patient's privacy, often is emotionally and financially costly, and places a personal decision in a public forum. However, particularly difficult cases may require judicial intervention, and policies should identify the types of issues that may require or benefit from legal counsel and court decisions.

The development of legislation on biomedical ethics has lagged behind the emergence of new dilemmas. Laws relating to a number of these issues vary significantly from state to state, and case law may often provide better guidance than statutes.

Implementation of Biomedical Ethical Policies

A heightened awareness of biomedical ethics must be supported by an emphasis on respect for patients and their families, respect among those working or volunteering in the hospital, and respect between employer and employees. In particular, the hospital should emphasize the importance of respect and consideration for categories of patients such as the aged, the noncompliant, and the poor.

Institutionwide educational programs are necessary to ensure that hospital policies and practices, their origin, and the reasons for them are clearly understood. Some hospitals also may wish to sponsor community forums or other programs to raise the community's awareness of these issues and how they are addressed in the hospital. Discussion of case studies* is one mechanism by which medical staff, other health care professionals, trustees, volunteers, and others can be alerted to the need for clear policies on biomedical ethical issues.

* See Use of Case Studies, Appendix B.

The hospital should maintain up-to-date resource materials on common biomedical ethical issues and make them readily available to employees, medical staff members, patients, and their families. Such materials ensure that consistent sources of information are available to all parties involved in a biomedical ethical decision or issue. Resources might include general articles on specific biomedical ethical dilemmas, information on state legislation that affects biomedical ethical decision making, and information concerning advance directives such as durable powers of attorney and living wills. Such resources might be developed jointly by several hospitals or with other community groups. The hospital ethics committee, if one exists, should usually develop educational programs and gather resource materials on ethical issues in patient care.

Using This Report

This report is intended as a guide for hospital administrators, trustees, medical staffs, nurses, and other health care professionals. It identifies issues that should be considered in resolving value conflicts that arise in delivery of patient care. Although it suggests approaches to resolving these conflicts, for the most part it avoids prescribing specific structures or policies. The committee believed that each institution should establish policies and processes appropriate to its size, resources, service mix, and mission.*

* See Recommended Areas for Hospital Policy and Practices Related to Biomedical Ethics, Appendix C.

Some biomedical ethical dilemmas are obvious and quickly become issues of discussion. Others are less obvious and are often woven into the fabric of a caring institution. Some volatile issues—do not resuscitate decisions, euthanasia, refusal of treatment, rationing—arouse public and professional concern. Others, however, relate to less obvious problems—how care can be provided and decisions can be made in an ethical manner. Issues such as confidentiality, restraints on patients, and safeguards for ethical decision making all fall into this category. This report attempts to deal with both obvious and less obvious biomedical ethical issues.

Because hospital size, scope of services, and mission are so varied, some parts of this report will not be equally helpful to all institutions. Sections on transplant procedures or highly advanced technological devices may have less relevance to the community hospital than to the teaching institution, but the comments in these sections also may be useful in more common decisions.

The committee recognized that the public policy issues regarding limits on access to health care services raise profound ethical problems that demand attention from the health care field as well as from society as a whole. However, because other AHA policy development bodies are examining these issues, the committee decided to focus its efforts on ethical issues related to patient care delivery in hospitals.

In this report the word *responsibility* usually means a moral or ethical responsibility. When the responsibility under discussion also is legal, specific mention is usually made of the legal requirement. The term *hospital* generally indicates the governing body, the administration, the medical staff, and others involved in establishing and implementing institutional policy. Ultimate accountability rests with the governing body.

Making Patient Care Decisions

* Although the term *physi-cian* is used, at times other health care professionals, particularly nurses, may be principals in the relationship.

Patient care treatment decisions are made in the context of the patient-physician* relationship and in the context of the health care setting. Decisions usually are made as part of an ongoing relationship, where both parties have agreed explicitly or implicitly on how decisions should be made. Whether the physician, patient, or both tend to take responsibility for decisions on medical care usually depends on the personality and preferences of both the physician and the patient and the severity of the condition or illness. Some treatment decisions, however, are of such magnitude and importance that a conscious attempt to ensure collaboration in decision making is warranted.

A key ingredient of collaborative decision making is open and truthful communication between the physician and patient. It relies on the physician's understanding and experience and the patient's self-awareness of personal values and goals. The physician provides information as completely and accurately as possible and makes recommendations for an individual patient that reflect sound medical judgment. The patient is encouraged to ask questions of the physician, seek information from other sources, and provide the physician with information and insights into personal preferences and lifestyle that can help the physician in recommending procedures and therapy. As a result, the decision is made collaboratively and agreed to by both parties. Of course, when a patient has a strong preference and expectation that the physician will assume the burden of decision making, this desire ordinarily should be respected. But the decision to have the physician be the decisionmaker should be made collaboratively.

Although the hospital does not have a major responsibility in this decision-making process, its policies should encourage ethical patient and physician collaboration. The hospital should have policies and practices that support and safeguard all aspects of informed consent and high-quality decision making, particularly because the hospital setting may complicate decision making. Patients often are in an unfamiliar and stressful environment that may impair their ability to make decisions and seek information; their reasoning and decision-making capabilities may be hampered by emotional factors associated with being sick or injured. In addition, they may lack the confidence and support derived from normal relations with family and friends and participation in daily routines.

Informed Consent

Informed consent is more than a signature on a standard form. Informed consent represents the patient's voluntary decision based on an understanding of the proposed action and its benefits, risks, and alternatives. The patient should have the opportunity to ask questions, request additional information, or consult with others as desired.

Consent is most often considered in terms of agreement to a particular procedure or to a set of routine procedures. Some hospitals ask patients to sign a general consent form for routine procedures and practices upon admission. An additional specific consent is usually required for surgery, other invasive procedures, or major diagnostic tests.

Although a patient may have signed a general consent form when admitted to the hospital, hospital staff cannot assume that the ethical and legal obligations implicit in informed consent have been met. Patients are entitled to information about tests, medication, and examinations that are part of routine care and treatment. In addition to indicating respect for the patient, discussing the purpose, process, and effects of routine procedures often results in greater cooperation from the patient and, in some cases, allows for patient refusal. Hospital policy should emphasize the importance of communication with the patient as to the purpose and effects of even routine patient care activities. Communication is even more important in larger hospitals where a number of persons may have responsibility for various aspects of the patient's care.

Hospitals have three major responsibilities in regard to informed consent. First, hospitals are responsible for assuring that proper informed consent has been obtained for diagnostic and therapeutic procedures performed at the hospital.

Second, hospitals should support and, if possible, develop education programs for physicians and the medical staff on effective ways to achieve ethically and legally acceptable informed consent. They may wish to encourage their medical staffs to develop guidelines to assist physicians in the communication process. Such guidance should emphasize the importance of communicating in a manner appropriate to the intellectual capabilities, knowledge, language, and emotional condition of the patient. In addition, it should stress the importance of objective and unbiased presentation of information, including the physician's recommendation.

Third, hospitals are responsible for making certain that patients are aware of their right to consent or reject proposed procedures and treatments. In addition, when possible, hospitals should assist patients who wish additional information or support in decision making. Hospital libraries or departments responsible for patient education may wish to have reading materials appropriate to laymen or to have cooperative arrangements with public libraries to obtain information for patients. In addition, a number of individuals such as chaplains, social workers, patient representatives, nurses, and others in the hospital may be able to provide information, counsel, and support for the patient in the decision-making process. If the patient agrees, information also may be shared with family members who may be involved in the process.

Patient Decision-Making Capacity

The ability to make a valid decision is essential to the patients' exercise of their right to participate in determining the course of their medical care and treatment. In most cases, there is little question as to the capacity or incapacity of the patient to make a valid decision. In others, however, the physical condition, effects of treatment, legal standing, intelligence, or psychological characteristics of patients may limit their ability to participate effectively.

Definition of Capacity. Decision-making capacity is the patient's ability to make choices that reflect an understanding and appreciation of the nature and consequences of one's actions and of alternative actions, and to evaluate them in relation to personal preferences and priorities. A patient's decision contrary to the physician's recommendation does not of itself indicate incapacity. Decision-making capacity is not synonymous with the legal term *competency*. A minor, who is legally not competent, for example, may possess considerable decision-making capacity, and a temporarily impaired adult who has not been legally declared incompetent may lack decision-making ability at a given time.

In the absence of indicators to the contrary, hospitals and health care professionals should assume that any adult patient has adequate decision-making capacity. A distinction should be made, however, between capacity to make some decisions and the capacity to make all decisions that may arise in the course of treatment. Even patients with limited capacity should be encouraged to make some decisions. Decision-making in the hospital extends beyond the dramatic life-death issues, to decisions on routine x-rays or tests and into such mundane areas as menu selection, preferences in clothes, decisions as to whether medication for pain is necessary, etc. Allowing the patient to make as many of these decisions as possible demonstrates respect for the patient and increases the patient's sense of autonomy. Furthermore, making these "mundane" decisions may well enhance the patient's capacity to make weightier choices.

In addition, some patients who lack the legal presumption of competency should be encouraged to participate in decision making about their own care. Some minors who have had a chronic disease for a long time, for example, often have substantial insights into the effects and desirability of various alternative courses of treatment. In addition, involving minors in decision making may increase their cooperation with the treatment regimen. Parents or guardians with legal authority to act on the minor's behalf should be encouraged to grant substantial deference to the minor's views.

Physicians, nurses, and other members of the health care team (including social workers, chaplains, patient representatives, or others involved in the care of the patient), as well as concerned family members, should be encouraged to identify what types of decisions an individual with limited capacity can make. Hospitals, through ethics committees, medical staff committees, publications, or in-service education programs, can enhance this process by further sensitizing those caring for patients to the importance of involving patients in various phases of decision making.

Assessment of Capacity. Although the attending physician has the principal responsibility to assess decision-making capacity, other members of the health care team and the patient's family and friends often may provide information and observations critical to evaluating adequacy of decision making capacity. The patient's nurse and support staff observe the patient's behavior. Family and friends can recognize if the patient is behaving abnormally, or expressing preferences that are discordant with longstanding values. Health care professionals, family, and friends should be encouraged to talk with the attending physician about observable changes that may affect a patient's capacity for decision making.

Decision-making capacity is judged against a lay rather than a professional standard. The question to be answered is whether the individual's ability to understand is within the acceptable range of what an average individual in similar circumstances might be expected to understand. The test[*] is how the individual functions in decision-making situations, rather than the particular category of patient—i.e., elderly, minor, mildly retarded, etc.

[*] See *Making Health Care Decisions, The Report of the President's Commission for the Study of Ethical Problems in Medicine and Biomedical and Behavioral Research*. Washington, DC: GPO, 1982.

In rare cases of strong disagreement about a patient's decision-making capacity among the physician, the patient, other health care professionals, and family and friends, consultation with appropriate specialists, such as psychiatric consultation, may be helpful or necessary. Such consultation may also be necessary to obtain a formal judgment of incompetence. It should be remembered, however, that assessments of a patient's capacity to make a decision apply to the immediate issue; they do not provide a long-term statement on the ability of the patient. In general, these assessments are informal, ongoing judgments to ensure that the decisions made reflect the preference and priorities of the patient.

As the patient's condition changes, decisions on capacity should be reviewed. If patients are capable of understanding information, they usually should be notified of concerns about their capacity and, if they desire, should be offered an opportunity for reassessment or access to institutional review mechanisms. Legal adjudication is also a possible alternative recourse for patients.

Barriers to Capacity. In some cases, the patient's ability to understand the nature and effects of treatment options is hampered by various barriers. For example, difficulty with the English language or hearing or visual impairments may prevent understanding. The hospital should see to it that, whenever possible, staff or volunteer interpreters are available; some states or areas have legal or regulatory requirements regarding interpreters. Medications or phases of illness that temporarily affect mental capabilities can be difficult to recognize and can limit the patient's capacity to understand the issues inherent in making a decision. Physicians should be encouraged to remove such barriers to decision-making capacity when medically reasonable and to consult with appropriate specialists, when necessary, to identify such situations.

In Cases of Incapacity. If a patient is considered to be incapable of making a particular decision, the patient's interests should be protected. Even this patient, however, should be included in the decision-making process to the extent possible. In these cases, usually the physician should make decisions in concert with a close family member or friend who acts as a surrogate.

Often the choice of appropriate surrogate is obvious—a spouse, another close relative, or a close friend, whose involvement throughout the course of treatment makes him or her the logical surrogate. In other cases, a patient may have specified, either through a durable power of attorney or a less formal communication, who should serve as a surrogate, if necessary.

The primary qualifications for the surrogate are that he or she be the person who knows the patient best, has been a close confidant, and can represent the patient's best interests.

The surrogate should cooperate with the physician and other members of the health care team to determine the patient's preferences about health care decisions. Information from living wills, durable powers of attorney, oral communications, other advance directives, and lifestyle commitments and preferences may provide information as to what the patient would have decided before decision-making capacity eroded. The physician, the health care team, and the family and friends should communicate and work together to make decisions that are consistent with the patient's known views or, if they are not known, with the patient's apparent best interests.

If a period of incapacitation is likely to occur as a result of illness, treatment, or a procedure, the attending physician should encourage the patient to discuss his or her treatment preferences before the care is undertaken. Such discussions could be undertaken with the physician, another member of the health care team, and/or an appropriate surrogate. Hospitals may wish to have information available to encourage patients to anticipate major decisions and document their preferences. In many states, a variety of legal mechanisms, including durable power of attorney, living wills, and natural death acts can assist in ensuring that the patient's views and wishes are respected.*

* See Living Will/Natural Death Acts, Appendix D, and Durable Power of Attorney for Health Care, Appendix E.

Although state requirements vary greatly, in most cases, court assessment of competency and/or appointment of a legal guardian is not necessary. However, the most common circumstances that alert hospitals and other parties to the possibility that court action may be advisable are when: (1) the incapacity is great and likely to be prolonged, and there is no obvious surrogate; (2) the capacity of the patient is questionable, and the decision to be made is significant; (3) the views of the surrogate are strongly at variance with medical judgment or the patient's known views; or (4) the choice of the individual to serve as surrogate is controversial and all efforts to resolve the matter at the hospital level have failed; and (5) family members radically disagree about the course of action in the case of a patient who lacks adequate decision-making capacity. The ethical imperative is protection of the patient's interests.

Treatment Selection

Many of the issues regarding selection of treatment are encompassed in the following policy and statement (pages 14-18) developed by the special committee and approved by the House of Delegates.

Patient's Choice
of Treatment Options

Policy

Health care decision making should be based on a collaborative relationship between the patient and the physician and/or other health care professionals who are primarily responsible for the patient's care.[1] The collaborative framework encourages communication, which contributes to sound decision making. Whenever possible, however, the authority to determine the course of treatment,[2] if any, should rest with the patient,[3] who may choose to delegate it. In the hospital setting, institutional methods should be established to reasonably assure that the patient may exercise this authority on the basis of relevant information necessary to make a sufficiently voluntary and informed decision. In addition, the health care institution should have methods to identify circumstances under which the patient's authority may be constrained and recourse to the judgment of others, including the courts, is appropriate.

Statement

The right and responsibility to select among treatment options presumes that the patient is capable of: (1) consulting with the physician[4] about and understanding the available treatment alternatives and their implications, and (2) making a choice. This process requires the patient's adequately-informed consent and may involve an evaluation of the patient's capacity to make a decision.

---

1) The term *physician* is used throughout the document, although other health care professionals may be responsible for or authorized to provide patient care.

2) For the purpose of this document, treatment can be interpreted to include diagnostic as well as therapeutic procedures.

3) For discussion of role of minors see "Role of Minors in Decision Making" on page 17.

4) Consultation might also take place with other responsible or authorized health care professionals involved in coordinating the patient's care.

This policy and statement was developed by the Special Committee on Biomedical Ethics, which had been established by the General Council in January 1983 to consider various aspects of biomedical ethical issues facing the health care field.
This document replaces the *Guidelines on the Right of the Patient to Refuse Treatment* that was approved in 1973. The House of Delegates approved the policy and statement in February 1985.

Collaborative Decision Making

Informed consent should reflect shared or collaborative decision making by the patient and the physician. The physician should provide information on the patient's condition, the recommended procedure and/or treatment with its significant benefits and risks, the significant alternatives for care or treatment (including no specific treatment), and the likely duration of incapacitation, if any.[5] Because patient understanding of this information is essential to informed consent, care should be taken to present it in language familiar to them. Although institutional policy should promote documentation of consent decisions, such documentation is evidence of but not a substitute for communication and understanding between patient and physician. Unless the physician believes the patient would object, it may be advisable and useful if this information is shared with the patient's family, which often is a valuable resource for both the patient and the physician. Health care institutions and professionals should see to it that patients have access to understandable information relevant to the treatment choices before them.

In cases where the patient has chosen to delegate the treatment choice selection to the physician or someone else, a discussion with the patient about the implications and ramifications of the treatment course to be pursued is still recommended. Often family and friends should be included in this discussion.

In some emergencies, obtaining voluntary and adequately informed consent may not be possible or may be detrimental to the patient's well being. In such cases, the patient's consent to the course of treatment chosen by a physician may be legally implied from the urgent circumstances surrounding the provision of that care.

Impact of Treatment Choice

The right to choose treatment includes the right to refuse a specific treatment or all treatment, or select an alternate form of treatment. If the patient decides to refuse all treatment, a written informed refusal is strongly recommended to protect the hospital, the physicians, and all other personnel from liability, if any, for failure to furnish treatment. This decision should also be documented on the patient's chart.

---

5) AHA *Policy on A Patient's Bill of Rights* [Appendix F].

If a patient chooses a course of treatment that is not accept-able to the attending physicians or other health care profes-sionals, those individuals may withdraw from the case, as long as doing so does not amount to legal abandonment. If a suitably qualified alternative physician or health care professional willing to comply with the patient's preference is available, transfer to the care of that individual should be offered to the patient. If no physician or qualified health care professional is willing to undertake the patient's choice of treatment, the hospital should have a policy to address what procedures relative to care of the patient should be followed. The hospital also should have a policy to help identify and address those situations when the course of treatment selected is unacceptable to the mission of the institution.

Laws regarding the right of a patient or someone on the patient's behalf to refuse treatment vary from state to state. Some state laws limit a patient's right to refuse treatment, and others make provisions to facilitate the exercise of this right. The hospital's and the physician's response to a refusal, whether action or nonaction, must be consistent with applicable law. If a refusal can potentially result in substantial detriment to the patient's health and well being, institutions should require that the appropriate administrative authority be informed. Protection of the patient's authority to select treatment at times may require either legal counsel or judicial proceedings.

Decision-Making Capacity[6]

Decision-making capacity is the ability to make choices that reflect an understanding and appreciation of the nature and con-sequences of one's actions. In health care treatment decisions, this is best understood as the patient's ability to understand the nature and effects of treatment options, and to appreciate the impact of a choice. Only when the patient's capacity to make decisions is definitely impaired and the effect of flawed decision making is potentially serious should the patient's right and responsibility for decision making be transferred to others.

When there is reason to doubt the usual presumption of ade-quate decision-making capacity, an assessment of capacity is made by the physician in consultation with the family, friends, and nurses and other health care professionals. The institution

---

6) Attention should be paid to the difference between decision-making capacity and legal competency. Decision-making capacity may exist, as in the case of a minor, where no legal competency exists. Legal competency may exist where decision-making capacity does not, as in the case of a temporarily impaired adult who has not been deemed legally incompetent.

Values in Conflict

should have effective policies to facilitate assessment of patients' decision-making capacity. The institution should have methods to ensure that the physician conducts these assessments when necessary. The hospital should also see to it that there are accessible and practical avenues by which concerns about a patient's capacity to make decisions may be raised by others, including family, friends, and nurses and other health care professionals. The hospital may also wish to have a policy under which a patient, in appropriate circumstances, would be informed both of any concerns raised by the assessment and of access to procedures for reassessment or to legal counsel. Only when the determination regarding decision-making capacity is controversial among concerned persons (including the patient) should legal guardianship proceedings be required.

When a patient lacks adequate decision-making capacity, substantial effort should be made to ensure that the choice of medical treatment is consistent with the known views of the patient. The decision makers must seek and take note of any information reflected in oral statements, life-style commitments, living wills, and so forth made by the patient before deterioration of decision-making capacity. These known views can sometimes be supplied by the family or an individual acting as surrogate. The surrogate should be a person or group of persons most likely to be able to advocate on the patient's behalf and to assess the patient's preferences and experiences. If the physician knows through informal communications, durable power of attorney, or living will of the patient's designation of a surrogate, that person should serve unless mitigating factors are apparent.

If the selection of the surrogate seems controversial, methods for institutional review and, if necessary, court adjudication, are required. In some cases, court appointment of a surrogate may be legally required. The institution should be prepared to refer difficult cases to court for guardianship determinations.

Role of Minors in Decision Making

Patients who are minors should be allowed to participate in decision making about their care to the extent possible with regard to their capacity to understand treatment options and outcomes. When a minor is deemed legally incapable of making a decision, that is, not considered to be a "mature" or "emancipated" minor according to state law, the parent or legal guardian usually will have the final decision-making authority. Mature or emancipated minors, as determined by state law, should be treated as adults with decision-making capacity.

Institutions should establish policies concerning the circumstances under which legal advice is to be sought for either the institution or the minor, including cases where a parent or guardian makes a decision that may be deemed adverse to the interests of a minor or opposed to the expressed views of a relatively mature minor.

Management Practices and Procedures

Hospitals have a responsibility to assess the effect of management practices and procedures on patient decision-making options and to foster awareness among health care professionals and key hospital personnel that some institutional practices necessary to ensure efficiency, such as some admissions or food service procedures, can unintentionally limit patient choices. For example, the patient often does not have the opportunity to make many of the routine choices in day to day living—when to have meals, wake up, have visitors, etc.

Documentation of Decision Making

Documentation of decisions regarding patient treatment promotes orderly procedures and more thorough consideration of options. Documentation also provides legal protection for and is often in the best interests of patients, patients' families, concerned health professionals, and hospitals.

Conclusion

The patients' role in determining the course of their medical treatment must be ensured in the institutional setting. Although these decisions should be made in collaboration with the attending physicians, the hospital must take a leadership role in ensuring institutional practices that support patients' decision making and in identifying when recourse to the judgment of others is necessary. ■

The Decision to Refuse Treatment. The right of the patient to refuse specific treatment or all treatment is widely recognized and upheld to various extents by state laws. The institution must facilitate the exercise of this right by patients who have decision-making capacity within the context of the mission of the hospital and society's stake in preserving the ethical integrity of the health care system and health care professionals.* The patient's refusal of all treatment should be made a matter of record to protect the hospital, involved physicians, and other personnel.

Forgoing Life-Sustaining Treatment. The patient's right to forgo life-sustaining treatment can be viewed as an extreme case of the patient's decision to refuse treatment. Ethically and legally the rights and protections grow out of the patient's right to choose or refuse treatment. Patients are entitled to refuse to seek or accept treatment or care for a condition or illness. However, a refusal certain to cause the patient's death can create ethical concerns when a patient or a patient's surrogate wishes to exercise this right within the hospital setting.

A number of factors must be taken into account by the hospital, including the views of the patient, legal requirements and ramifications, the perspectives of the medical staff and other members of the health care team, the hospital's mission, and the corporate responsibility for high-quality health care. When these factors cannot be satisfactorily reconciled, patients who wish to discontinue or not to initiate life-sustaining treatment or care are often put in an adversarial role in relation to the hospital and physician, and the courts may be required to serve as the mediator or decision maker.

Whenever possible, decisions should be made at the level closest to the patient—between the patient and the physician, or between the family of a comatose or otherwise mentally incapacitated patient and the physician. Hospitals, however, should offer support from other health care professionals involved in the patient's direct care, including, when appropriate, the staff nurse, involved house staff, hospital social worker, patient representative, and chaplain. On another level, an ethics committee could provide additional guidance. Recourse to a

* Courts have varied in their approach to balancing patients' rights with those of the hospital and society in general. Generally, four societal interests are identified: (1) preservation of life not in a terminal condition, (2) prevention of suicide, (3) protection of innocent third parties, and (4) effect on the integrity of health care professionals and on other members of society. See, e.g., *Bartling v.Superior Court,* 2 Civ. No. B007907 (2nd App. Dis., Calif. 1984); *Bouvia v. County of Riverside; Riverside General Hospital* No. 159780, Sup. Ct. Cty. of Riverside (Dec. 16, 1983), *Superintendent of Belchertown State School v. Saikewicz,* 370 N.E.2d 417 (Mass. 1977); *In re Storar,* 52 N.Y.2d 363, 420 N.E. 2d 64, 438 N.Y.2d 266, *cert. denied,* 454 U.S. 858 (1981); *In re Colyer,* 6760 P.2d 738 (Wash. 1983).

court ruling should be reserved for those cases in which the patient or surrogate prefers court procedures or the issues resist resolution at a less formal level.*

Decisions related to the patient's right to refuse life-sustaining treatment should be consensual and result from information sharing and discussion among the attending physicians, other involved health care professionals, and the patient or the patient's family. Self-interests of family, friends, and health care professionals should not be allowed to compromise pursuit of the patient's best interests.

Do Not Resuscitate Decisions

Do not resuscitate (DNR) decisions are concerned with whether resuscitation is appropriate in terms of the patient's overall condition and personal values. A DNR decision may be legally, ethically, and/or medically appropriate. Because a decision not to resuscitate is a decision not to prolong life through an available form of technology, it has been a subject of great concern in our society, which has placed a high value on extending life.

As part of its commitment to high-quality patient care, each hospital should have policies addressing when, how, and by whom DNR decisions should be made and documented. Because of differences in state laws, hospital missions, and hospital and medical staff bylaws and rules, no one DNR policy or set of policies is appropriate for all hospitals. Development of DNR policies, however, can be an educational process for the institution that further sensitizes the medical staff, nursing staff, administration, and trustees to the ethical dimensions and ramifications of such decisions. It should be strongly emphasized that DNR orders are not inconsistent with maximum therapeutic care and in no way indicate that the course of treatment should be changed. Guidelines on DNR, such as those developed by the Medical Society of New York State* may be useful in development of DNR policies.

Participation in the Decisions. Efforts to reach a decision on resuscitation should be made in advance of the acute episode—a cardiac or respiratory arrest—in cases when it is likely to be appropriate. In the absence of a specific directive not to resuscitate, normal resuscitation procedures should be undertaken. Therefore, a DNR decision requires advance discussion and communication between the physician and the patient or a surrogate.

Values in Conflict

Although attending physicians must determine if resuscitation is likely to provide any medical benefit to the patient, they should not make these decisions in isolation. If the patient is capable of making a decision, a DNR order should result only from collaborative and consensual decision making. If a patient does not agree to the proposed DNR order, it should not be written.

If the patient does not have the capacity to participate in the decision, an appropriate surrogate should be involved. The physician also should consult with other health care professionals caring for the patient—nurses, house staff, etc.—as well as involved family members. This consultative process should involve extensive information gathering concerning the medically relevant details of the patient's condition as well as observations about the patient's attitudes and desires.

In some cases, patients have an opportunity for self-determination and expression through advance directives such as living wills or through informal communications with physicians, family members, or friends. In other cases, particularly when the acute episode has not accompanied a prolonged or chronic illness, patients may not have exercised such opportunities to make their views known. If the surrogate and the physician do not agree, mechanisms for institutional review, such as an ethics committee, should be available.

The three essential elements guiding the decision whether or not to give a DNR order should be: (1) maximum medical data; (2) preferences of the patient, interpreted if necessary by the patient's family or other surrogate; and (3) consultation among physicians, health care professionals, and family members. A DNR order should never be written without the knowledge of the competent patient or the family of or surrogate for the patient.

Documentation and Implementation of the DNR Order. To ensure clear direction, DNR decisions should be recorded as formal orders by attending physicians. The progress notes should reflect discussions about the DNR decision with the patient, family, and health care professionals caring for the patient, as well as the relevant data contributing to the decision.

The attending physician is responsible for making certain that the DNR order is discussed with other members of the health care team caring for the patient. DNR orders and the reasons for them should be communicated to all shifts of health care professionals caring for the patient. Hospitals should have mechanisms to make certain that the DNR decisions are regularly reviewed and withdrawn when the patient improves and has a better prognosis. Other implementation considerations include whether members of the house staff or nursing staff may refuse to cooperate with a DNR order and, if so, how they can exercise this option without disrupting or compromising* patient care.

* See The Hospital and Health Care Professionals—Moral Prerogatives and Limits, page 36.

Some hospitals also might wish to make a distinction between cardiac or respiratory arrests that occur during medical intervention as opposed to those that may occur from natural causes. The issue in these cases is whether some diagnostic or therapeutic procedure rather than natural causes brought on the arrest. In these cases, because reversibility is more likely and the complication probably was not discussed in advance, resuscitation might be highly appropriate even though a DNR order to cover other circumstances has been written.

Caring for Patients

The way in which the hospital and health care professionals care for and relate to patients is a major part of the ethical environment of the hospital. Interactions on virtually every level among and between hospital employees, health care professionals, patients, and their families have ethical components. It would be impossible for this report to discuss every aspect of relationships affecting hospital operations and procedures. This section, however, highlights some of the major ethical issues involved in providing care to patients: maintaining confidentiality, using restraints, providing continuity of care, disclosing errors and negative outcomes, identifying problems of professional competence, establishing ethics committees, and assuring the moral prerogatives of the health care institution and health care professionals.

Confidentiality

* See *Policy on A Patient's Bill of Rights,* Appendix F.

Patients have the right to expect that all communications and records pertaining to their care will be treated as confidential.* Hospitals have a legal and moral responsibility to establish institutional mechanisms and practices to protect the confidentiality of patient information and limit access to patient records to the fullest extent possible. Confidentiality can be viewed as a quality of communication—or as it has been defined, as "a process of communicating in a relationship of trust." Since the earliest practice of medicine, the privacy of patient information has been a foremost tenet. Despite this long tradition of confidentiality, changes in the environment of the hospital, laws and regulations, and activities of third-party payers are affecting the range and type of information deemed confidential.

Much confidential patient information often is available to many in the hospital at the touch of a computer button. This information may be needed for reimbursement, evaluated by peer review committees, and shared freely among the various specialists in medicine and the allied health care fields who care for a particular patient. Because patients must share with physicians and other health care professionals information about personal habits, history, and circumstances relevant to their health or illness, the hospital must develop policies that protect and support a climate conducive to confidentiality and clarify when strict confidentiality may be overridden. Issues such as the use of patient information in education and research should be considered, and policy should stress that the duty of confidentiality is unchanged if a patient's care is subsidized by public funds.

To ensure a climate of confidentiality, all those in the hospital should be informed of and understand the hospital's practices concerning access to and use of patient information. To enhance this climate, the hospital might want to establish nonpublic areas specifically for discussion of cases among the health care team.

The right of the patient to request or sanction disclosure of otherwise confidential personal information takes precedence over the hospital's obligation to protect it. When practicable the hospital should help patients understand their option to limit the scope of the information to be disclosed to the minimum necessary. In signing consents for release of information to insurers and others, patients may not be aware that they may restrict disclosure to specific types of information for specific purposes. When it appropriately discloses information to others, the hospital should emphasize that the information is confidential and that the receiving party is expected to maintain its confidentiality. A signed and notarized document to such an extent may be required by both parties. Patients also have the right to view their own confidential records and to have misinformation corrected, except as controlled by state law.

Also subject to state law, confidentiality may be overridden when the life or safety of the patient is endangered, such as when knowledgeable intervention can prevent threatened suicide or self-injury. In addition, the moral obligation to prevent substantial and foreseeable harm to an innocent third party usually is greater than the moral obligation to protect confidentiality. Protection of the interests or rights of the public as a whole also overrides the obligation of confidentiality. Common examples of public interests, as defined by state laws, include child abuse or mental illness posing a danger to society. In addition, hospitals, physicians, nurses, and others have legitimate legal duties to report certain communicable

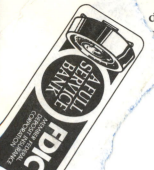

diseases, injuries, and other conditions to public health officials or other appropriate authorities.

The American Hospital Association *Policy on A ...tient's Bill of Rights** sums up the issue from the ...atient's perspective:

> The patient has the right to every consideration of his privacy concerning his own medical care program. Case discussion, consultation, examination, and treatment are confidential and should be conducted discreetly. Those not directly involved in his care must have permission of the patient to be present. The patient has the right to expect that all communications and records pertaining to his care should be treated as confidential.

Restraints on Patients

Use of physical or chemical restraints requires a judgment as to whether the risks to the patient or others outweigh the obligation to respect the autonomy and self-determination of the patient. Although this issue is prominent in literature pertaining to psychiatric services, it usually has not been widely discussed in relation to general hospitals. Restraints are, of course, most frequently used in the best interests of the patient's health and safety. However, it is possible that they may be used in a hasty manner for management convenience when alternatives might have been better for the patient. Because the potential for abuse of restraints is great, hospital policies should address the ethical use of restraints, including bed side rails, safety vests, tranquilizers, wrist restraints, etc.

A hospital's policy on the use of restraints should cover who is entitled to authorize restraints, appropriate use of restraints, timely review of decisions to use restraints, and procedures for administering and monitoring the use of restraints on patients. When developing these policies, hospitals should consult with their legal counsel because state laws differ on authorization for restraints. Some states require written authorization from the physician and/or provide for emergency situations.

Particular attention should be paid to the role of the nurse, who is usually the health care professional applying restraints and most affected by their application. Nurses should be encouraged to discuss the use of restraints for particular patients with attending physicians, and hospitals should have procedures to follow when nurses and physicians do not agree on appropriate action and when potential danger to the patient or others is a factor. Hospitals should provide in-house educational programs for nurses and other interested health care professionals on how to assess the need for restraints and possible alternatives to their use.

Policies should highlight those circumstances that may result in misuse or abuse of restraints. The impact of staffing patterns on use of restraints should be studied, although it should be recognized that even reasonable staffing levels may not allow the type of care and attention that would eliminate the use of restraints. Confusion and agitation may justify restraints, but they also may be symptoms of other problems; and the use of restraints should not replace identifying and, if possible, resolving the problems.

Although some practices, such as use of side rails or postoperative restraints, provide routine protection for patients, frequent use of more restrictive restraints, particularly when they are an indignity to the patient or could cause physical or psychological damage, should be used only as a last resort. Furthermore, because chemical restraints may impair the patient's ability to participate fully in decisions about treatment, their use should be carefully scrutinized. (See also Barriers to Capacity, p. 11.)

Policies should specify the frequency with which decisions to use restraints should be reviewed and should provide guidance on the following:

- Documentation of the types of behavior requiring use of restraints
- Appropriate communication with the patient and the patient's family about the need for restraints
- Documentation of a decision by a patient with adequate decision-making capacity, or a patient's surrogate, regarding use of a restraint
- Proper fitting of a physical restraint or titration of a chemical restraint to minimize the risk of harm to the patient
- The frequency with which physical restraints should be checked and removed and chemical restraints reassessed to ensure maximum patient safety, comfort, and freedom

Continuity of Care

As a result of growing awareness of the limits on health care resources, acute inpatient services—the most expensive form of health care—are being deemphasized. For health care institutions, this creates new questions. Does the hospital's role in relation to its overall care for patients end with their discharge? Does the hospital have an obligation to patients after they have left the hospital? Does the hospital have any additional responsibility for patients if the community has not provided for a continuum of health care apart from the hospital? What role does the hospital play in the continuum of care?

The answers to these questions are complex and focus attention on the obligations of the hospital to its patients and its community. The hospital is seldom in the position —either in terms of mission or finances—to meet the community's entire spectrum of health care needs. However, important and vital roles other than as direct provider are open to the hospital, and the hospital has a moral obligation to do what it reasonably can to facilitate continuity of care for patients upon discharge from the institution.

Continuum of Health Care. The hospital as a center for health care in the community is usually able to identify gaps or inadequacies in health care services. Staff, particularly discharge planners and social workers, are well equipped to provide information on nonacute health care programs that would benefit the community. If the hospital— because of its mission, priorities, or financial resources— cannot provide a needed service, it should call the community's attention to that need and attempt to work with other health and social service organizations to meet it.

For example, hospitals serving an aging population should be particularly alert to the needs of older patients following discharge for home health programs, day care, respite care, homemaker services, meals on wheels, and/or telephone check-in programs. Whenever such services are established, the hospital necessarily plays a coordinating role in transfer arrangements. Under most circumstances this includes a moral responsibility to accept a readmission if the medical condition of a transferred patient deteriorates and acute care again becomes a necessity.

Hospitals also should be alert to the need for specialized programs for categories of patients, such as hospice programs for the terminally ill. However, patients should not be channeled automatically into particular types of alternative care programs and should be made aware of their option to change their decisions. As in all treatment decisions, patients should have the opportunity to make fully informed choices.

Discharge Planning. The American Hospital Association *Guidelines on Discharge Planning** are helpful in defining the process of finding appropriate nonhospital care and treatment. That document describes the purpose of discharge planning: "to ensure the continuity of high-quality patient care, the availability of the hospital's resources for other patients requiring admission, and the appropriate utilization of resources." Among the most essential elements discussed in the guidelines are several of particular relevance to care for the elderly or the dying: early identification of patients likely to need complex posthospital care; patient and family education, assessment, and counseling; and postdischarge follow-up. The importance of discharge planners being knowledgeable about care alternatives in the community cannot be overemphasized.

* See *Guidelines on Discharge Planning,* Appendix H.

Medical Errors and Negative Outcomes

The way a hospital deals with errors in care and negative outcomes has significant ramifications for its ethical relationships with its patients and community. Negative outcomes and errors can include nosocomial infections, conditions that are side effects of other treatment regimens, treatment errors, etc. Hospitals and health care professionals must acknowledge that some negative outcomes and even errors are inevitable and that they may occur under conditions ordinarily associated with good results. Such acknowledgment is an important element of professionalism and conducive to the sharing of information and the progressive reduction of error to a minimum. The institution should create an environment that makes such candor possible. A good risk management program combined with the educational activities of an ethics committee can help create a hospital atmosphere in which health care professionals are encouraged to report both negative outcomes and errors.

The normal reaction to a negative outcome or a medical error should be full disclosure to the patient or the patient's surrogate. Timely disclosure to and prompt communication with patients and their families can greatly mitigate the impact of negative events and outcomes. Disclosure should include what happened; the causes, if known; and any known effects on the patient's short-term and long-term health. Partial disclosure restricts the patient's autonomy. A position that partial or non-disclosure serves the patient's well-being requires careful scrutiny to determine if it could be a response to a conflict of interest. Delays or cover-ups are neither morally nor legally acceptable alternatives; they violate respect for the patient and increase the vulnerability of institutions.

The hospital and the physician should make an effort to distinguish between significant and insignificant errors in patient care and respond appropriately. For example, administering a medication an hour late may have no appreciable effect on the patient, but an accidental surgical severing of a nerve that may permanently or temporarily deprive the patient of feeling in a part of the body requires positive action and full disclosure.

Provider Competence

Although mistakes and negative medical outcomes are a part of health care delivery, patterns of practice and care that suggest incompetent, illegal, or unethical activities should not be accepted. The hospital has an ethical and legal responsibility to make certain that the health care provided by its employees and by physicians and others with hospital privileges meets acceptable standards. Tissue committees, quality assurance programs, review of credentials, and utilization review all play a role in detecting problems related to the competency of various health care professionals. Beyond these programs, hospitals should create an environment that provides maximum protection for patients from incompetent, illegal, or unethical practices. In some cases, hospitals and many health care professionals also are legally required to report to appropriate professional and/or state authorities unsafe or unethical practices, particularly those that have not been eliminated or corrected through earlier efforts.

This hospital concern extends to all patient care activities, whether conducted by an independent physician with admitting privileges, a physician employed by or under contract to the hospital, a hospital employee, or a volunteer. Hospitals should encourage their medical staffs, employees, and volunteers to recognize when the patient care practices of others present a danger to the health or safety of patients and to make certain that appropriate steps are taken to rectify the problem. Hospitals should have clearly defined, publicized, and easily accessible mechanisms for receiving, investigating, and taking action on disclosures and allegations of unethical behavior or incompetence by health care professionals. These mechanisms will vary depending on hospital organizational structure and size, but it should be remembered that direct reporting to supervisors of such problems may be unrealistic in some cases. The hospital must create a system that protects the rights of all parties—the individuals who disclose information, the involved health care professionals, and the patient.

Hospitals should have mechanisms to ensure that patients have a known method of voicing concern about what they perceive to be unsafe or unethical practices in the hospital. Patient information materials should identify who should be contacted with concerns about care. Patient representatives, ombudsmen, social workers, chaplains, or administrators may all be appropriate contacts for patients. Although some patient concerns may be based on a lack of understanding of medical procedures and hospital routines, the observations may help identify patterns of questionable care. Patient reporting of concerns gives health care professionals an opportunity to correct problems as well as to explain procedures that may be misunderstood by or disturbing to patients.

Creating an atmosphere conducive to prompt and appropriate disclosure puts the hospital and those who work there on record as not tolerating practices and continued performance that are below standard. To achieve this perspective, the hospitals' efforts must be thorough and confidential, and provide responsive, timely investigation and corrective action.

Ethics Committees

There is a strong temptation to view ethics committees as the new "quick fix" to the biomedical ethical dilemmas confronted in health care. Ethics committees, however, are not a new phenomenon. They have existed under other names in many health care institutions, particularly church-related hospitals, for some time. Although such committees hold promise for assisting patients, their families, and health care professionals to make decisions, they are not a panacea for all problems nor do they remove the hospital's responsibility for the care it provides or replace the traditional decision makers in health care.

The Guidelines on Hospital Committees on Biomedical Ethics (p. 33-35) address a number of general issues to be considered in development of such comittees including their function, composition and deliberations. Several aspects of such committees were not directly addressed in the guidelines but discussion of them may be useful to hospitals as they develop or review the progress of ethics committees. They include the effect of confidentiality requirements on the way in which a committee is structured and functions, access to the committee, and the purview of the committee.*

* See Legal Issues and Guidance for Hospital Biomedical Ethics Committees, Appendix I.

The importance of confidentiality raises a number of issues, including the role, if any, of community representatives on ethics committees, the need for patient consent, and the committee's position in the hospital structure. Although community representation on a committee that develops educational programs and provides forums on biomedical ethics is probably a positive force, such representation on a committee that will have access to confidential patient information, in most cases, should be approached with caution. If such representation is considered vital, the hospital could require an individual not professionally bound to confidentiality to sign a standard oath of nondisclosure or have patients or surrogates sign a consent form to allow the release of necessary information to an ethics committee.

Seeking the concurrence of the patient to have a case brought to an ethics committee often may be advisable, particularly if the committee includes individuals external to the hospital. Such concurrence, however, should not be required if it would prevent physicians and other health care professionals from seeking advice and guidance. The hospital should communicate its practices regarding use of ethics committees to patients in its patient information materials.

In some hospitals, particularly public institutions, confidentiality is a factor in determining the place of the committee in the hospital structure. For example, if records of administration or governance committees are subject to public disclosure, then establishing an ethics committee as a medical staff committee (with multidisciplinary membership) would be a better way to ensure confidentiality.

Everyone involved in the hospital—medical staff, nurses, other employees, trustees, volunteers, patients, and patients' families—should have access to the ethics committee as a resource, with the committee chairman or another involved individual acting as the gatekeeper. In its advisory capacity, it should be open to those seeking counsel about the range of ethically acceptable responses to a conflict of values.

Patient care issues should be the first priority for hospital ethics committees, although some hospitals also may want ethics committees to look at broader issues such as cost and access as they relate to patient care. Some caution should be used, however, to avoid overburdening committees or detracting from their patient care orientation. There is a danger that a concern for broad institutional dilemmas could influence ethical judgment on individual issues. When there are ethics committees in more than one hospital in a community, the committees may find it productive and efficient to work together to provide educational programming for the community or to develop self-education programs for their own members.

Hospitals should also recognize that although the patient's financial considerations might be taken into account by an ethics committee in its overall efforts to identify the range of ethically acceptable alternatives in a given situation, hospital financial issues should not be a foremost consideration for ethics committees; nor should an ethics committee be asked to play the role of de facto rationer of health care services on a patient-by-patient basis.

Guidelines

Hospital Committees on Biomedical Ethics

This guideline document is intended to provide general advice to the membership of the American Hospital Association, as approved by the General Council.

Introduction

The growth of medical knowledge and the rapid expansion of medical capabilities and technology have generated unprecedented opportunities and challenges in the delivery of health care. At the same time, this growth and expansion have created increasingly complex ethical choices for physicians, health care professionals, patients, and the families of patients. Recent efforts to clarify biomedical ethical issues on the institutional level have focused on the use of hospital biomedical ethics committees. Such committees, sometimes called "ethics committees," "human values committees," "medical-moral committees," or "bioethics committees," hold promise for identifying the ethical implications of these problems and their possible resolutions, if they are established with a clearly defined purpose and an understanding of their capabilities and limitations.

Institutional ethics committees are one of several approaches to address medical ethical matters. If an institution chooses this approach, the following guidelines may assist in determining the organization, composition, and function of these committees. Because such committees are relatively new and largely untested, the guidelines are not intended to be prescriptive or directive.

The American Hospital Association's General Council created a Special Committee on Biomedical Ethics in 1982. This multidisciplinary committee prepared these guidelines as part of its charge to assist hospitals in developing institutional processes to deal with the educational and decision-making challenges presented by biomedical ethical issues. These guidelines were approved by the AHA General Council on January 27, 1984.

Functions

Although institutional ethics committees may have one or more functions, they seem particularly suited to: (1) directing educational programs on biomedical ethical issues, (2) providing forums for discussion among hospital and medical professionals and others about biomedical ethical issues, (3) serving in an advisory capacity and/or as a resource to persons involved in biomedical decision making, and (4) evaluating institutional experiences related to reviewing decisions having biomedical ethical implications. Ethics committees should not serve as professional ethics review boards, as substitutes for legal or judicial review, or as "decision makers" in biomedical ethical dilemmas. An ethics committee should not replace the traditional loci of decision making on these issues.

Educational programs on biomedical ethics issues serve to heighten awareness and provide guidance on identification of cases where ethical problems may arise. Such programs may be offered to medical staff, the hospital staff, and the community. Forums for the discussion of these issues serve similar purposes by providing an opportunity for physicians, nurses, administrators, trustees, clergy, ethicists, and others to consider and discuss a number of diverse perspectives.

The use of ethics committees in an advisory role to assist physicians, other health care professionals, and patients and their families to make decisions when confronted with dilemmas is probably their most complex function. Ethics committees often may make recommendations at the request of an attending physician, another hospital professional closely connected with the case, the hospital administration, and the patient or the patient's family. Access to the committee should be open to all those involved in patient care decisions. Hospitals should design and implement systems to bring to the committee's attention certain kinds of issues and to address similar issues in a reasonably consistent manner.

Composition

The members of an ethics committee should be selected in keeping with its objectives and represent a range of perspectives and expertise. It may be multidisciplinary and may include physicians, nurses, administrators, social workers, clergy, trustees, attorneys, ethicists, and patient advocates (representatives).

Hospital legal counsel should be available at the request of the committee, and legal review of its recommendations may be necessary.

To be most useful and effective, an ethics committee should be a standing committee, and its members should be approved by the appropriate authority within the institution. This structure provides continuity and enhances the credibility of the committee. It also provides an opportunity for the committee to develop an understanding of the permissible range for discretion and latitude within which biomedical ethical decisions may be made. The committee should meet regularly and whenever necessary to provide advice and recommendations. As a general rule, no one who is personally involved in the case in question should serve on the committee while the case is being considered.

Deliberations

Issues that may be brought to an ethics committee acting in an advisory capacity should relate to patient care.

If a recommendation is made by the committee, it should be provided as appropriate to the physicians, nurses, and other health care professionals involved in treatment, and should be offered to the patient and the patient's family or other surrogate.

The confidentiality of patient information and the patient's privacy should be respected. The circumstances under which documentation of the committee's recommendations should appear in the patient's medical records should be determined by each institution with the advice of legal counsel.

The manner in which the committee considers an issue or a particular case should depend on the individual circumstances. The committee may review and discuss materials submitted to it, or it may meet with the health care team involved and others as needed, including persons acting on the patient's behalf.

Conclusion

Each institution should take the steps necessary to implement suitable mechanisms that will reasonably provide for sound decision-making practices and for responsible and timely assessment of medical and ethical issues. ∎

The Hospital and Health Care Professionals— Moral Prerogatives and Limits

Health care providers—individual health care professionals and institutions—also have justifiable claims to self-determination and autonomy. Although, in great part, this report has emphasized the need for a hospital environment conducive to ensuring respect for the patients' self-determination and autonomy, some attention to the moral prerogatives of the hospital and health care professionals is warranted.

Hospital Prerogatives. The hospital corporation through its governing body represents a set of values to the community. The hospital's moral commitments to its community are generally embodied in the statement of its mission. Each hospital has the prerogative to develop a mission reflecting its historical roots and philosophy.

* See also p. 39.

Every hospital must make decisions concerning its service mix,* that is, decisions on the range of services it will provide. These decisions usually relate to perceived community needs for a service, the consistency of the service with the hospital's mission, the availability of the service elsewhere, the hospital's ability to provide the service, and the financial viability of the service. Even to the extent that a service may be needed and consistent with the hospital mission, the hospital's moral prerogative to maintain its own fiscal viability makes financial issues a legitimate consideration. This is not to say that hospitals should provide only services that are financially attractive; the hospital has the obligation to make honest and sincere efforts to provide needed services and to develop alternative mechanisms to subsidize unprofitable but necessary services.

In exercising these prerogatives, the hospital should be responsive to the community's need to understand the hospital's mission, the services it will not offer because of conflict with its mission, and those services it cannot offer because of various limitations. In the selection of service mix, the self-determination of the institution may come into conflict with the self-determination of the patient. If the hospital has chosen not to provide a service, the patient may not have convenient access to it. Hospitals should be prepared to facilitate transfer of patients to other health care institutions that offer different services, if the patient so desires.

Values in Conflict

Professional Prerogatives. Health care professionals also have moral values and the right to embody these values in their professional activities. Hospitals should make every effort to accommodate the moral convictions of health care professionals. However, health care professionals also must be sensitive to the purpose of the health care institution and acknowledge that others may not share their personal convictions. To balance the responsibility of the hospital to its patients and its employees and to balance the employees' obligation to patients and to themselves, employees must inform their supervisors of convictions that may affect their performance under particular circumstances. To the extent possible, the hospital should seek to accommodate employees who object to participating in certain procedures by ensuring that other personnel will be available to provide the necessary care and treatment or, in some cases, to refrain from treatment. The hospital should not allow the patient's care to be compromised because of internal conflicts.

Hospitals should be sensitive to the emotional strains that health care professionals may feel as a result of their patient care decisions and activities. Hospitals have an obligation to make policies related to biomedical ethics clear so that the demands and limits on employees are fully understood, and that employees are able to work with guidance on appropriate behavior related to biomedical ethical issues.

Deciding on Services

Rapidly expanding medical capabilities combined with increasing demands to contain health care costs are raising difficult ethical questions concerning resource allocation within the hospital. Lack of national or regional policies or guidance for allocating scarce and costly resources places a de facto responsibility on health care providers to develop policies to guide decisions on service mix, use of new technology, organ transplantation, and rationing.

Service Mix

Selecting the mix of services appropriate to a hospital's mission and resources is an ongoing process requiring systematic and periodic evaluation, which takes into account other community resources as well as customs and traditions. For example, whether a hospital establishes a home care program or an outpatient clinic, it must weigh alternatives, examine the relationship of the service to existing services, and determine the number of patients likely to benefit from the service. A decision to discontinue an existing service must be subject to the same process.

Service-mix decisions should be made collaboratively by hospital executive management, trustees, and medical staff. If appropriate, the decision-making process may involve community representatives such as business and labor leaders, the clergy, coalition representatives, educators, and local government officials.

Continued pressures for cost-effective management require hospital executives and governing boards to eliminate excesses and effect economies wherever possible, without threatening the quality of patient care. Some hospitals may be forced to make decisions about curtailment of services for which adequate payment is no longer available. At this point the business functions and the healing ethics of the hospital may come into conflict. Obviously, some compromises will be necessary. To continue services without regard for their business implications would be fiscally irresponsible; to pursue business practices without regard for service access and outcomes would be morally reprehensible. Hospital boards and executives are obligated to reconcile such dilemmas.

Discontinuation of a service sometimes may be in the best interests of both the institution and its patients, because it may permit the hospital to use its resources in ways that better serve the community. If a hospital perceives a community need but cannot justify providing a new service or continuing a low-volume service, it should encourage exploration of alternatives, including affiliation and/or sharing services with other institutions. Sharing pharmacy, x-ray, or similar services, or joint investments in or cooperative leasing of mobile service units, for example, may in some areas be the most cost-effective way to provide needed care.

New Technology

Policies relating to new technology must be consistent with the hospital's mission. Typically, even the most promising new technology presents many unknowns regarding costs, safety, efficacy, and efficiency. To the extent that these may be quantified and projected, the hospital should make reasonable efforts to assess them based on available data and, where possible, on the known experience of other institutions. Practices regarding technology must be based on how acquisition will affect the hospital's ability to provide existing services, other facilities in the community, how many individuals will benefit, and how the technology may affect the safety and comfort of patients. Once new technology has been acquired, these factors provide the basis for periodic evaluation and for decisions as to whether to continue providing the service. Before acquiring new technology, the hospital must be certain that its professional staff has the qualifications and competence to properly apply it.

Acquisition of new technology often requires a trade-off between the new and exciting and the more basic. The ethical implications of these trade-offs must be considered. Although major new technology increases the hospital's prestige, this should not be a primary reason for acquiring new equipment. Moreover, because hospital acquisition of high-priced equipment often generates public interest, it may require special attention to privacy and confidentiality for patients.

The way in which cost-effectiveness is considered in technology decisions varies according to the mission of the institution. Teaching and research hospitals involved in testing innovative equipment, drugs, and new procedures, for example, would balance the cost-effectiveness issue differently than would a community hospital. Not all technology is expensive to purchase, but even inexpensive items may result in new procedures and practices that have implications in terms of cost, quality of care, exclusion of other services, and human resources, and these should be thoroughly assessed.

Organ Transplantation

In the last 25 years the range of transplantable organs has grown to include corneas, kidneys, bone marrow, skin, lungs, livers, endocrine glands, and hearts. During the past decade, improved surgical techniques, better tissue matching, and the use of new immunosuppressive drugs all have made transplants more feasible. As a result, many institutions are pressured to decide whether transplantation services are appropriate for the hospital and its community.

When making these decisions, the hospital should rely essentially on the same principles as for acquisition of other new technology. Particular attention should be given to the impact of this type of resource allocation on the hospital's ability to meet the more common health care needs of its community, and to the regional need for the transplant program.

Equally critical in transplant service decisions is whether the institution can procure an adequate supply of organs in an ethically acceptable way and is prepared to make distribution decisions on available organs and costly transplantation procedures. Although decisions about which patients are to receive organs are often made on an ad hoc basis, in most situations, priority should be placed on candidates who are most likely to significantly benefit from transplant procedures.

Rationing of Services

Discomfort with the concept of health services rationing is widespread in the United States, but the rationing or limiting of services by hospitals is likely to increase as technology proliferates and demand for scarce resources increases. The federal government confronted this issue in regard to renal dialysis when it made dialysis available to all rather than establish a rationing system. Although this approach is inconsistent with the government's current intention to limit increases in health care spending, it reflects the unwillingness of policymakers at all levels to deal with the rationing issue. The hospital, however, must address it in regard to its services and community.

No hospital can be expected to provide what it does not have. However, the institution should periodically review its allocation of resources to determine if their use best meets community needs.

Generally, a hospital may refuse to provide a service to a patient if the procedure is inappropriate to its mission (for example, therapeutic abortion, artificial insemination). The hospital also may refuse to provide services to a patient requesting an elective procedure or one beyond its capability, such as open-heart surgery. Refusal to provide services that are critical to the well-being of the patient, however, is not acceptable solely or primarily because the patient is unable to pay for care, and the hospital should make every effort to assure fair and compassionate distribution of its available resources. The hospital should make every effort to provide nonemergency as well as emergency services to medically indigent patients. The hospital also has a community service responsibility to help provide services to patients considered socially "difficult" (for example, chronic drug abusers, custodial patients, alcoholic patients, prisoner patients, or noncompliant individuals who nevertheless return repeatedly for care). Depending upon their missions and financing, hospitals deal with such situations differently; however, they share in the community's responsibility to assist individuals in need of care.

Very costly procedures, usually involving sophisticated technology, are most likely to raise questions about rationing. Often such rationing is implicit, such as in use of beds in intensive care or specialty care units, or in the assignment of "interesting" or unusual cases to the most prestigious specialists. To the extent possible, hospital leadership—the governing board, executive management, and medical staff—should recognize such implicit rationing so that its ethical implications can be better understood and addressed.

Thinking about the Future

The challenge of dealing with biomedical ethics in hospitals grows more complex as the dilemmas become more difficult. This report has attempted to provide guidance to help hospitals develop policies and procedures to resolve the ethical questions that arise in delivery of patient care. Although the form of these policies and procedures will differ, they must stress two elements: awareness and communication. Heightening the awareness of everyone in the hospital concerning the ethical dimensions of patient care and encouraging open communication concerning policies, incidents, and problems relating to ethics are essential to an effective institutionwide approach to biomedical ethics.

Hospitals and those concerned with public policy will face major questions that have significant biomedical ethical components in the coming years. For hospitals, the need to compete in the health care marketplace will bring major issues to the fore—including reevaluation of missions, difficulty in cooperating with competitors, ethically sound advertising, and the need for cost-efficiency versus the need for a service that is not cost-effective. Assuring appropriate services for the increasing number of the elderly, who have greater needs for support and custodial services, will require hospitals to evaluate their responsibilities in promoting or providing such services. Greater fiscal restraints will force many hospitals to reevaluate their allocations of resources for research, teaching, and patient care.

Hospitals will have to remain sensitive to the stress that health care professionals feel as a result of their involvement in biomedical ethical conflicts and dilemmas and to intensify efforts to ensure that their ability to function does not become impaired by physical, emotional, and/or intellectual fatigue.

For society and those concerned with public policy, many of the questions will be more fundamental: How should access to health care be assured and who should pay for it? How can society be assured that advances in medical science and research will be applied wisely—for example, genetic engineering? When does prolongation of life become prolongation of dying? What are the implications of a shift from publicly funded to privately funded scientific research? What responsibility should individuals have for the consequences of their harmful lifestyle decisions? How much of funding should be allocated for health care as opposed to other essential needs? What amount of total health care dollars should be expended on research and prevention as opposed to direct patient care?

None of these questions will be easily answered, but they cannot be ignored. Hospitals cannot be passive in the face of such dilemmas. They must work individually, together, and through their associations to resolve institutional and community-level issues. They must take the lead in drawing national attention to issues that should be discussed and debated openly in the broadest public policy arenas.

Dealing with the differing values inherent in biomedical ethical issues is a never-ending process for hospitals and health care professionals. As medical knowledge continues to expand, social priorities and emphases continue to shift, and individuals continue to raise fundamental concerns about the ethics of health care treatment and delivery, hospitals will need policies and procedures to guide resolution of biomedical ethical questions.

It is the moral responsibility of each hospital to recognize and respond to issues that raise such questions. Certainly much remains to be done. This report is an attempt to provide a framework to increase awareness and to stimulate discussion of biomedical ethical issues in the hospital.

Appendix A

**Roster of the American Hospital Association
General Council Special Committee on Biomedical Ethics**

Chairman

Paul B. Hofmann, Executive Director, Emory University Hospital, Atlanta

Mr. Hofmann has been in hospital administration for 18 years in Georgia, California, and Massachusetts. He is a fellow in the American College of Hospital Administrators and served as chairman of the AHA Council on Research and Development. He is currently an AHA representative to the American Medical Association Health Policy Agenda for the American People project. He has written numerous articles on such issues as health care for the hospitalized elderly, hospital costs, and the role of computers in hospitals. He received a bachelor's degree and a master's degree from the School of Public Health, University of California, Berkeley.

Vice-Chairman

Christine I. Mitchell, R.N., Clinical Specialist-Staff Development and Research, The Children's Hospital, Boston

Ms. Mitchell has had experience as a clinical nurse, an assistant professor of nursing, and a counselor. From 1979 until 1981, she was a Kennedy fellow in ethics and did consulting on ethics in nursing at schools of nursing and at the Kennedy Institute. She has given numerous lectures and presentations on the issue of ethics and was associate producer of *Code: Grey,* a film on nursing ethics. She received bachelor and master of science degrees in nursing from Boston University and a master's degree in theological studies from Harvard University.

Members

Stanley S. Bergen, Jr., M.D., President, University of Medicine and Dentistry of New Jersey, Newark

Dr. Bergen has been president of the University of Medicine and Dentistry of New Jersey since 1970. Prior to that he was senior vice-president for medical and professional affairs for New York City Health and Hospitals Corporation and chief of community medicine at Brooklyn-Cumberland Medical Center. He serves on the executive committee of the board of the Hastings Center and currently is involved in study groups concerning death and dying and the use of drugs in sports. He received his bachelor of arts degree from Princeton University and his medical degree from the College of Physicians and Surgeons, Columbia University.

Bob L. Bybee, Administrator, Palo Duro Hospital, Canyon, Texas
Mr. Bybee has been a hospital administrator for 10 years and has been active in the Texas Hospital Association as a district adviser and a member of the THA house of delegates. He has had training in family, group, and individual counseling and in child care and geriatrics. He has a bachelor of science degree in religious education from Howard Payne University. He has also studied business and marketing at Texas Tech University and purchasing management at the Kellogg Center at Michigan State University.

Robert M. Cunningham, Jr., Health Care Writer and Lecturer, Chicago
Mr. Cunningham's career as a writer and lecturer on hospital subjects spans more than four decades. A former editor of *Modern Hospital,* he has been an editorial consultant to the Blue Cross and Blue Shield Association and a contributing editor of *Hospitals* and *Trustee* magazines. He is the author of a number of books on health care subjects, including *Governing Hospitals, Asking and Giving,* and *Wellness at Work.* He is a graduate of the University of Chicago and is an honorary fellow of the American College of Hospital Administrators.

Dorothy J. Danielson, R.N., Howard Young Medical Center Corp., Minocqua, Wisconsin
Mrs. Danielson has had considerable experience in clinical nursing, quality assurance, nursing education, and administration. She is a past president of the American Society for Nursing Service Administrators. She received her bachelor of science degree in nursing from Boston University and her master of science degree in nursing from Columbia University. She is currently establishing a hospice program at Howard Young.

William G. Gordon, Administrator, St. Luke's General Hospital, Bellingham, Washington
Mr. Gordon has been a hospital administrator for 15 years. He has served on the board of trustees of the California Hospital Association and has been on the board of direc-

tors of the Hospital Council of Central California. He is currently a member of the AHA House of Delegates and is a member of the American College of Hospital Administrators. He has a bachelor of science degree in business administration from Fresno State University and a master's in business administration from Golden State University.

Joanne Lynn, M.D., M.A., Assistant Clinical Professor, Division of Geriatric Medicine, George Washington University Medical Center, Washington, DC

In addition to her teaching, Dr. Lynn is medical director of the Washington Home and Hospice. She served as assistant director of the President's Commission for the Study of Ethical Problems in Medicine and Biomedical and Behavioral Research. A fellow of the Hastings Center, she has written extensively on biomedical ethical issues. She earned a medical degree from Boston University, a master of arts in philosophy and social policy from George Washington University, and a bachelor of science degree from Dickinson College.

Kenneth A. Marshall, Chairman, Board of Trustees, Deaconess Health Services Corporation, St. Louis

A former vice-president of Sherwood Medical Company, Mr. Marshall was in the hospital supply business for 35 years and has been a leader in the Health Industry Manufacturers' Association, serving as its chairman in 1979. He is active in the Hospital Association of Metropolitan St. Louis and is vice-chairman of the board of trustees of Deaconess Hospital, St. Louis. He has a bachelor's degree from the Massachusetts Institute of Technology and completed the Harvard Graduate School of Business advanced management program.

Richard A. McCormick, Professor of Christian Ethics, Kennedy Institute of Ethics, Washington, DC

Rev. McCormick is the Rose F. Kennedy Professor of Christian Ethics at the Kennedy Institute of Ethics at Georgetown University. He has written a number of books and articles on ethical issues. He is a past president of the Catholic Theological Society of America and a fellow of the Institute of Society, Ethics and the Life Sciences (Hastings Center). He is an adviser on ethics to the Virginia Hospital Board-International Children's Hospice and a past member of the former Department of Health,

Education and Welfare Ethics Advisory Board. He has bachelor and master of arts degrees from Loyola University in Chicago and a doctorate in theology from the Gregorian University in Rome.

Marcella L. O'Halloran, Hospital Trustee, Waterville, Maine

Mrs. O'Halloran has been involved in hospital governance on the institutional, state, regional, and national levels for 25 years. She is currently a trustee at the Mid-Maine Medical Center and is the Maine delegate to the National Congress of Hospital Governing Boards. She was a member of the steering committee for the First National Conference of Women Health Care Leaders on Cost Containment. She has a bachelor of arts degree from Colby College.

John A. Reinertsen, Executive Director, University of Utah Hospital, Salt Lake City

Mr. Reinertsen has been a hospital administrator for 30 years in Illinois and Utah. He has been active in metropolitan, state, and national hospital association activities. Most recently, he served as vice-chairman of the AHA General Council's Special Committee on Federal Funding for Mental Health and Other Health Services. He has a bachelor's degree from Augustana College in Rock Island, IL, and a master's degree in hospital administration from Northwestern University, Evanston, IL.

Seymour Siegel, Professor of Ethics and Theology, Jewish Theological Seminary, New York City

Prof. Siegel currently serves as executive director of the U.S. Holocaust Memorial Council. He has been a professor of humanities in medicine at the Medical College of Pennsylvania and a visiting professor of religion at Carleton College, Georgetown University, Union Theological Seminary, and several other universities. He was a senior research fellow at the Kennedy Institute and served on the President's Commission. Rabbi Siegel has bachelor and master of arts degrees from the University of Chicago and a baccalaureate and a doctorate of Hebrew letters from the Jewish Theological Seminary of America.

Mark Siegler, M.D., F.A.C.P., Associate Professor, Department of Medicine, University of Chicago

Dr. Siegler is chief of the general medicine section and director of the Center for Clinical Medical Ethics at the

University of Chicago—Pritzker School of Medicine. He is the author (with Jonsen and Winslade) of *Clinical Ethics.* He is a Fellow of the Hastings Center and serves as a consultant on ethical issues to the American College of Physicians. He serves on the editorial board of the *American Journal of Medicine,* the *Archives of Internal Medicine,* the *Journal of Medicine and Philosophy,* and the *Bibliography of Bioethics.* He has a bachelor of arts degree from Princeton University and a doctor of medicine degree from the University of Chicago. His clinical training included a chief residency at the University of Chicago and a fellowship as senior registrar in medicine at the Royal Postgraduate Medical School in London, England.

William B. Spofford, Religious Coordinator, St. Luke's Regional Medical Center, Boise, Idaho

Bishop Spofford has 25 years of experience in clinical pastoral education and has served as a hospital trustee. He has been chief chaplain at Massachusetts General Hospital in Boston and McLean Hospital in Belmont, MA. Prior to working at St. Luke's he was at the Diocese of Washington (Episcopal Church). He is a founding member of the National Association of Social Workers. He has a bachelor of arts degree in sociology from Antioch College; a bachelor's degree in theology from the Episcopal Divinity School, Cambridge; and a master of social work degree from the University of Michigan's School of Social Work.

Staff

Richard L. Epstein, LL.B., Counsel to the Special Committee, Senior Vice-President, American Hospital Association, Chicago

Mr. Epstein is senior vice-president of the American Hospital Association and is responsible for the AHA's legal affairs, directing all litigation and legal activities in which the Association is involved, and supervising the AHA Office of the General Counsel. He has also been an AHA group vice-president and senior general counsel. From 1970 to 1978, he served, by appointment of the President, as a member of the Federal Services Impasse Panel, which mediates labor cases involving unionized federal government employees. He received his bachelor of arts degree from Amherst College and his law degree from Yale Law School.

Edward W. Weimer, Secretary, Special Committee on Biomedical Ethics

Mr. Weimer has been an AHA staff member since 1960 and has held various positions, including regional director, director of the Division of Administrative Services, and assistant director of the Association. He currently is an assistant secretary of the AHA as well as director, Division of Conventions and Meetings. In addition, he has served as a consultant on a variety of advisory committees of the U.S. Public Health Service. He has a bachelor of arts degree from Colorado State College and a masters in business administration from the University of Chicago.

Michael Lesparre, Assistant Secretary, Special Committee on Biomedical Ethics

Mr. Lesparre is director of the Division of Communications and Public Relations, Washington office of the AHA. He was previously director of the Association's New York office, which at the time was the office for AHA Region 2. He has served as staff to numerous AHA committees and is currently co-secretary to the AHA Council on Allied and Government Relations. He has a master's degree in journalism from Northwestern University.

Gail M. Lovinger, Assistant Secretary, Special Committee on Biomedical Ethics

Ms. Lovinger is project manager in the American Hospital Association Office of the Secretary. She was previously associate manager of policy communication in the AHA Division of Public Affairs. She has assisted in staffing several AHA policy development and governance bodies. She has a master of arts degree in speech communication from the University of Illinois, Champaign-Urbana.

The special committee gratefully acknowledges the contributions of various AHA staff members not assigned to the special committee, particularly William Read, Ph.D., Mary Ahern, J.D., and Alexandra Gekas. The special committee also gratefully acknowledges the work and support of the Legal Task Force on Biomedical Ethics of the AHA Office of Legal and Regulatory Affairs and the AHA Academy of Hospital Attorneys.

Appendix B

Use of Case Studies

Case studies are an excellent way to sensitize groups to the ethical issues in patient care and the need for hospital policies on them. They are a valuable learning tool for any group within the hospital, particularly for ethics committees in the early stage of development. They also can benefit health care professionals, support personnel, volunteers, and trustees, as well as interested groups within the community.

Case studies can be used in a number of ways, depending on the size and composition of the group. For example, large groups can be divided into several small groups, all of which discuss and recommend action on the same case study. The various recommendations are then compared and discussed by the whole group. As an alternative, several different case studies can be used for a large subdivided group. It also may be productive to choose a "blue ribbon" panel to play the role of an ethics committee examining a case and have the audience observe the discussion.

Case studies are usually most useful when individuals of different backgrounds and professions are participating, particularly physicians who can discuss the medical indications in the case, trustees, patient care nurses, administrators, clergy or chaplains, and attorneys.

Attached are several case studies that may be useful. These cases should be adapted to the circumstances that most closely fit the hospital. Hospitals may find it useful to develop their own case studies, and suggested guidelines for developing case studies follow.

1. Determine goals of the case study

2. Develop a case that:
* Requires a heightened awareness of biomedical ethical ramifications
* Could occur in your hospital
* Demonstrates the need for additional education

- Demonstrates the lack of clear guidelines
- Involves a conflict

3. The case study should include:
- Relevant background information on major parties
- Description of involved parties (patients, family, friends, physicians, nurses, other health care professionals)
- Description of condition and prognosis
- Description of relevant past course of treatment or care
- Description of the health care setting
- Information about relevant state laws
- The same type of information that would be available to the persons involved in resolving the problem.

4. Develop questions for discussion, such as
- What ethical principles are involved?
- What types of policies would help guide the decision?
- Who should be involved in making the decision?

Case Study 1*

Sharon Rose is a fourteen-year-old girl who was initially admitted to Community Hospital nearly two years ago with a three-week history of chest pain and progressive shortness of breath on exertion. It was noted on admission that she appeared thin and undernourished with height and weight more than two standard deviations below the mean for her age group. A chest X-ray revealed opacification of the right chest and a mediastinal shift to the left. After one liter of serosanguinous fluid was removed from her chest, a large anterior mediastinal mass became evident by X-ray. The fluid drawn from her chest contained lymphoblasts and lymphocytes. After further studies, the following diagnoses were made:

* Reprinted with permission of David Thomasma, Ph.D., Loyola University, Chicago.

(1) malignant lymphoma, lymphoblastic type—involving the mediastinum, right pleural cavity, and right supraclavicular nodes
(2) undernutrition
(3) idiopathic seizure disorder

Sharon has remained in initial complete remission for sixteen months now, and she has been treated on an outpatient basis for fourteen of these months.

One week ago she was admitted to the hospital again for cough, fever and fatigue. She was found to have diffuse pneumonia of the left lung, for which she has been given antibiotics and supportive measures. Her admission hemoglobin of 7.3 Gm% has progressively declined to 4.4 Gm%, however; and her condition is deteriorating rapidly.

The physicians treating Sharon judge that a blood transfusion is now essential if there is to be any hope of saving her life. However, her parents remain adamant in their refusal of transfusion—and Sharon herself indicates that she agrees with their decision.

Sharon was given chemotherapy and radiation therapy with a rapid and complete tumor regression. During the next four months, Sharon suffered moderate toxic side effects—including anemia, weight loss, oral ulceration and radiation pneumonitis—requiring a hospitalization and modification of chemotherapy dosage.

The management of these problems was complicated by the parents' refusal to permit blood transfusions on religious grounds. They were Jehovah's Witnesses. Their wishes in the matter were honored—especially since it was not thought that the blood transfusions were absolutely essential for effective management.

Suppose you were one of the physicians treating Sharon. What should you do?

1. Honor their wishes and withhold the blood transfusion. Make Sharon as comfortable as you can while nature takes its course.

2. Send in a social worker to investigate the family dynamics and the strength of their convictions about refusing blood transfusions.

3. Initiate studies to determine whether the malignant lymphoma has returned or whether this pneumonia is from an independent source.

4. Initiate court proceedings to authorize transfusion against the wishes of the patient and her family.

You chose to send in a social worker to investigate the family dynamics and the strength of their convictions about refusing blood transfusions. After lengthy individual interviews with each of the parents and Sharon, the social worker files this report:

Sharon Rose is a fourteen-year-old girl whose cognitive, emotional, and personality development all appear to be within normal limits.

Sharon has had a troubled family situation. When she was two years old, her natural father—Ted Rose—left the home—at her request, according to the report of Sharon's mother (whose name is Lilly). Lilly filed for divorce about a year later, and Ted did not contest the action. Shortly after the divorce was granted (with Lilly given sole guardianship), Ted moved to another state. Lilly reports that Ted has never visited Sharon nor made any direct contact with either of them since that time, although the court-mandated child-support payments are transmitted (sporadically) through Ted's sister who lives in the city.

When Sharon was seven, Lilly married again; but the marriage lasted less than a year and was apparently stormy throughout. At the divorce hearings, Lilly accused her second husband of physical abuse towards both herself and Sharon, as well as sexual abuse of Sharon. However, the judge pointedly commented in the divorce decree that no evidence was introduced to support the latter charge.

Between marriages, Lilly supplemented the meager and sporadic child support payments by working as a waitress at the sandwich counter of a local drugstore. She reports that her income was insufficient to provide for the needs of her and her child. "I made just too much to draw welfare, but too little to pay all the bills," she says.

Until she married Bill Stone (her present husband) when Sharon was ten, Lilly recounts that neither she nor Sharon had been active in any church. But Bill has been a Jehovah's Witness all his life; and, since her marriage, both she and Sharon have become extremely active in the local Jehovah's Witness congregation.

Neither Lilly nor Sharon appear to have much understanding of the rationale behind the Jehovah's Witness objection to blood transfusions. One gets the strong impression that the primary interest of both is in honoring Bill's deep convictions—Lilly in order to preserve her marriage and Sharon out of respect and affection for Bill's kindness and warmth as her step father.

Given this information, what should you do?

1. Honor their wishes and withhold the blood transfusion. Make Sharon as comfortable as you can while nature takes its course.

2. Initiate studies to determine whether the malignant lymphoma has returned or whether this pneumonia is from an independent source.

3. Initiate court proceedings to authorize transfusion against the wishes of the patient and her family.

*Reprinted with permission
of David Thomasma, Ph.D.,
Loyola University, Chicago.

J.B. was an 81-year-old active and alert man who was actively engaged in his business and the development of a recreational camp for the physically disabled, this latter interest stemming from his elder son's disability from polio which left him unable to walk. On routine physical examination, he was found to have a prostatic nodule, for which a transperineal needle biopsy was performed. During the next several hours, the patient became febrile and hypotensive. A leukocytosis and thrombocytopenia developed with peritoneal signs. A diagnosis of septic shock and an acute abdomen secondary to ischemic bowel was made. The relative risks of operating versus not operating in a case of presumed small bowel infarction were discussed with the patient and family, and an operation was readily agreed upon.

At celiotomy, a dusky left colon was discovered which extended below the peritoneal reflection. The mesenteric arteries were pulsatile and venous thrombi were not noted. The decision was made not to resect the ischemic colon, a colostomy thus being avoided, and the patient was closed and treated with vasodilators postoperatively. During the next few days, he had rectal bleeding and mucosal sloughing requiring transfusion, confirming the diagnosis of ischemic colitis. By the fourth postoperative day, the patient was off cardiac support and vasodilators and tolerating a clear liquid diet.

On the fifth postoperative day, he began to experience more respiratory depression associated with poor expectoration. A chest x-ray demonstrated bilateral pneumonia and pulmonary edema. Systemic antibiotics were begun. His respiratory rate continued to increase throughout the day, and by evening was 40-50/minute. Arterial blood gases at that time revealed a pH of 7.38, pO2 42 torr. and pCO2 54 torr. He was electively intubated at this time. The patient was extubated eight days later with normal arterial blood gases and ventilatory capabilities.

After extubation, the patient stated that he had a living will, and he now requested that no further heroics be done to save his life, including re-intubation should that become necessary. He had been alert and oriented for the last eight days since surgery. During that day, he became increasingly unable to handle his secretions, became febrile again, increased his respiratory rate to 40/minute and became hypercarbic and hypoxic. Re-intubation was recommended, and the patient refused. His family was

Values in Conflict

divided regarding whether to re-intubate their father, and two family members who believed he should be intubated contacted the patient's lawyer. The lawyer insisted that the patient be ventilated, and informed the family that this was the only responsible course of action.

Case Study 3

Married retired federal employee, 68 years old. Terminally ill with leukemia and mentally incompetent due to course of illness, bedridden, needing total care including intravenous feeding. Being kept alive by periodic and regular blood transfusions (Type O positive). Recently admitted to the hospital from a nursing home due to complications of pneumonia, which is being successfully treated. With aggressive treatment and care and continuing blood transfusions, can be kept alive for at least six months.

Wife: 65 years old.
Son: 44 years old, married with children, lives nearby.
Son: 42 years old, single, lives out-of-state.

Patient has a personal physician who has known the patient for the last 20 years.

Patient has adequate hospital coverage and physician coverage through private insurance (no Medicare). Limited long-term care benefits and personal resources being used to pay for nursing home care (SNF level).

Patient has told wife before onset of confused and weakened state that he does not want to be kept alive by artificial means, or his life prolonged if he can no longer function independently. Children and physician know his wishes, but eldest son believes that stopping transfusions would be murder. Wife and other children want treatment stopped. Nurse administrator of the patient's unit known to oppose withdrawing treatment.

Hospital

Rural, small, 100 beds. Private, non-profit, non-denominational.
Community = 17,000.
Hospital serves a population area of 25,000.
Patient's physician is on staff (one of eight physicians using hospital).

Questions

1. Who needs to be involved in the decision on withdrawing treatment?

2. What hospital policies should be in force to help guide high quality appropriate decision making?

3. What steps might the hospital go through in the decision making process?

4. What might be the role of an ethics committee in this case?

5. What additional information would be helpful in addressing this specific case?

6. What further questions with regard to consideration of such cases should be raised?

Case Study 4*

* Reprinted with permission of Program on Human Values and Ethics, University of Tennessee, Center for the Health Sciences, Memphis, Tennessee.

R. B. was 15-year-old-boy, the only child of parents now in their 50s. He was a sophomore in high school, academically above average, and interested in sports, having earned positions on both the football and track teams.

His present illness began early in September, when he injured his right leg in football practice. In the next two days after that injury, he continued to have pain just below the knee of the right leg. After two days of continued pain, the coach recommended whirlpool baths but felt that he could continue practice. The pain continued for another week in spite of this program and he mentioned it to his father, who said that he probably had a bruise and that it would improve. However, the pain persisted for still another week, and at that time the football coach called the parents and recommended that he be taken to the family physician for further studies. The parents were able to get an appointment toward the end of the next week and the family physician found local tenderness and some swelling. He obtained a roentgenogram at the local hospital and the following day asked the parents to come to his office for a discussion. At that time he told them that it looked as if there was a tumor in the bone just below the right knee. Because of these findings, he referred the patient to the St. Jude Children's Research Hospital.

On further study at this institution, the boy was found, indeed, to have a tumor in the right fibula which was interpreted as being most likely osteosarcoma. There was no evidence of tumor involvement in the lungs or in the bones. The rest of the physical and laboratory findings supported the impression of clinically localized osteosarcoma. A recommendation of an above-the-knee amputation of the right leg was made, to be followed by a period of adjuvant chemotherapy according to the current protocol study, lasting for a period of 10 to 12 months. The protocol study included randomization to receive or not receive immunotherapy with irradiated tumor cells during the course of treatment.

The parents and the boy were understandably upset about this proposal. The boy in particular was concerned about the amputation and asked if there were alternative methods of treatment. He told the parents he did not want to have the leg removed and would refuse treatment. His parents were undecided but finally went along with the boy's wishes. In spite of long conversations, the parents remained adamant. It was recommended that they return home, talk with their family physician, family, and pastor about this decision. After an additional week of discussion and continued contact with this hospital, the decision was finally made to allow amputation and treatment.

The amputation went without incident, and the boy was fitted immediately with a walking prosthesis. Chemotherapy, according to protocol, was begun after receiving permission from the boy and the parents. After 4 months, however, the boy decided against any further chemotherapy. He had lost his hair with treatment and had episodes of vomiting, especially in association with the administration of methotrexate. He was missing school and was particularly concerned and distressed about the fact that his friends were beginning practice for track. In talking with both parents, the physicians had been able to convince the father of the need for continued treatment but the mother said that she would not allow any further treatment if the boy did not want it. The boy had expressed to her his conviction that he had been cured and needed no further treatment. The father reluctantly concurred with the mother about this decision, although it was clear that actually he had withdrawn from the situation shortly after the initial surgery and it was the mother who was truly determining the response to the son's decision.

Case Study 5*

* Reprinted with permission of Program on Human Values and Ethics, University of Tennessee, Center for the Health Sciences, Memphis, Tennessee.

J. P. was a sixty-year-old black male with an admittedly sketchy past history due to ineffective follow-up. However, he was apparently diagnosed as having chronic renal disease, secondary to hypertensive renovascular disease, approximately 3 years prior to his last admission. During the 9 months prior to this admission, the patient had been hospitalized four separate times for management of his renal disease and associated medical problems.

Throughout his known contact with the health care system, the patient had expressed and demonstrated a certain disregard for recommended therapeutic modalities. He refused to be compliant with a diet, intermittently took prescribed medicines, and almost consistently missed appointments. His laissez-faire approach to his chronic disease was interrupted only when his family brought him to emergency rooms for acute problems—GI distress, profound weakness, lethargy, and even seizures.

With the progress of his renal disease, the option of dialysis was discussed with him and he usually refused with apparent understanding of the implications. However, during the last of these four hospitalizations, he tentatively agreed to peritoneal dialysis in the future if it meant saving his life. Nevertheless, soon thereafter the patient was brought to the emergency room again with significant metabolic derangement and still refused dialysis. He was treated symptomatically before being released.

On his last admission, the patient was a lethargic, incoherent, severely wasted individual with physical findings consistent with uremia, including a pericardial friction rub. Laboratory examination revealed the presence of metabolic acidosis with severe derangement of AM electrolytes, anemia, and evidence of a urinary tract infection with possible sepsis. The patient was unable to discuss therapeutic options and the family could not be reached. Contact was made with a neighbor, who confirmed that the patient had not been compliant with his complicated pharmacological regimen of at least ten different agents. Apparently, the patient had progressively deteriorated since his discharge 8 weeks earlier.

Values in Conflict

Case Study 6*

* Reprinted with permission of Susanne Durburg, R.N., Evanston Hospital, Evanston, IL

Mrs. D. was a 40-year-old diabetic admitted to the hospital for bilateral amputation of both legs below the knee. She has been on dialysis for approximately nine years. She lives alone and up until the present has been able to maintain independent function. Her nephrologist has asked for a psychiatric consultation since Mrs. D. has discussed with him her desire to forgo surgery and stop dialysis.

Mrs. D. discussed her concerns with the psychiatrist on three different occasions. She recognized her prognosis was poor and expressed appropriate fear of the consequences of her decision to cease dialysis. However, she was more fearful of the likelihood of her loss of independence if she had surgery, while only delaying her deterioration and death. In the psychiatrist's judgment, Mrs. D.'s responses to her situation were realistic and she was judged to be capable to make a decision. She was not suffering a clinical depression.

Subsequent to his visits with Mrs. D., the psychiatrist met with the staff and the patient's attending physician. Together they outlined a plan of care for Mrs. D., which included termination of dialysis with the expectation of subsequent coma and death. A plan was outlined, whereby the staff would maintain Mrs. D.'s comfort throughout this final ordeal.

Appendix C

Recommended Areas for Hospital Policy and Practices Related to Biomedical Ethics

Issue	Policy*	Practices	Page References
Allocation of Resources, review of		X	41-42
Collaborative Decision-Making	X		7-22
• Informed Consent	X	X	8-9
• Capacity, barriers to		X	11-12
• Capacity, assessment of	X		10-11, 16-17
• Role of Minors	X		9-10, 17
Confidentiality	X	X	23-25
Continuity of Care		X	27-28
Do Not Resuscitate Decisions	X		20-22
• Institutional Review, surrogate-M.D. disagreement		X	21
• Review of DNR decisions		X	22
Forgoing Life-Sustaining Treatment, support for patient, family		X	19-20
Medical Errors		X	28-29
Moral Convictions of Employees, accommodation of		X	36-37
Provider Competence		X	29-30
Restraints	X	X	25-26
Service Mix Selection		X	39-40
Technology Acquisition	X		40-41

* Policies related to biomedical ethics should:
  • be consistent with the institution's mission
  • be the basis for conflict resolutions regarding values
  • be sensitive to community standards
  • be the basis for educational programs
  • respect the patient's responsibility for decision making
  • support the appropriate roles of others in decision making
  • support an environment of information-sharing and consultation on ethical questions
  • respect personal liberties
  • support conflict resolution at the level closest to the patient.

Appendix D

Living Will/Natural Death Acts

Statutory Citations

Alabama Natural Death Act, Ala. Code secs. 22-8A-I-10 (1981).
Written declaration required; signed in presence of two disinterested witnesses who must be at least 19 years old. Declaration form in law, but may include personalized instructions. Invalid during pregnancy. Physician must be notified of document's existence, make it part of medical record. In effect until revoked; may be revoked at any time. Immunity to physician, health care professional and facility for good faith compliance with declaration. Compliance with declaration or transfer of patient required. Criminal penalties for concealment or falsification.

Arkansas Death with Dignity, Ark. Stat. Ann. secs. 82-3801-3804 (1977).
Written declaration required, executed with same formalities as required for execution of a will. Minor or adult mentally or physically incapacitated may have form executed by another, e.g., parent, spouse, guardian, as specified in statute; must contain signed statements by two physicians. Immunity from liability for person, hospital or other medical facility acting in compliance.

California Natural Death Act, Cal. Health & Safety Code secs. 7185-7195 (1976).
Written declaration required; signed in presence of two disinterested witnesses. Form in statute must be followed. Patient in skilled nursing facility cannot execute directive unless one witness is state-appointed advocate. Invalid during pregnancy. Revocation at any time. Effective for five years. Immunity from civil or criminal liability for physician, health facility, and licensed health professional acting under physician's direction. Declaration valid if executed after terminal diagnosis, but if not can be given weight as evidence of patient's wishes. Physician must comply with directive or arrange transfer, or will be guilty of unprofessional conduct. Criminal penalties for certain acts of falsification or concealment of a directive.

Delaware Death with Dignity Act, Del. Code Ann. tit. 16 secs. 2501-2509 (1982).

Written declaration; signed in presence of two disinterested witnesses. Invalid during pregnancy. Adult by written declaration may appoint agent who may accept or refuse treatment. Revocation at any time. Declaration to be made part of medical record. Effective for 10 years. Resident in nursing home or related institution must have declaration witnessed by special state-appointed advocate. Immunity from civil and criminal liability for physician, individual acting under physician's discretion, and health facility for good faith compliance. Criminal penalties for falsification or concealment.

District of Columbia Natural Death Act of 1981, D.C. Code Ann. secs. 6-2421-2430 (1982).

Written declaration, signed in presence of two disinterested witnesses. Physician to be notified of declaration and to place in medical record. Form in statute but modifications allowed. Patient in intermediate care or skilled nursing facility may execute declaration if one witness is state-appointed advocate. Revocation at any time. Patient's desires always supercede declaration. Physician must comply or transfer, or commit act of unprofessional conduct. Immunity from civil and criminal liability for physician, health care professional, health facility or employee. Criminal penalties for falsification or concealment.

Florida Life Prolonging Procedure Act, Fla. Stat., ch. 84-58, secs. 765.01-.15 (1984).

Written declaration, witnessed by unrelated persons. Oral declaration signed in declarant's presence. Physician to be notified of declaration and make it part of medical record. Form in statute but may be modified. Revocation at any time by any method. If no declaration, withholding or withdrawal of life-prolonging procedures from incompetent adult may occur if consultation and written agreement between physician and certain specified individuals, e.g., spouse, guardian, parent, witnessed by two persons. Physician refusing to comply must transfer. Invalid if pregnant. Immunity from civil or criminal liability for health care facility, physician or person acting under physician's direction for compliance. Criminal penalties for falsification or concealment.

Values in Conflict

Georgia Living Wills Act, Ga. Code Ann. secs. 31-32-1-12 (1984).
Written declaration signed in presence of two disinterested witnesses. Form prescribed in statute if declaration made while patient in hospital or skilled nursing facility must also be witnessed by medical director or medical staff chief. Revocation at anytime. Effective for seven years. Invalid during pregnancy. Immunity from civil or criminal liability for physician, person acting upon his/her direction, hospital, skilled nursing facility and any agent or employee for good faith compliance. No person civilly liable for failure to comply; unwilling physician to discuss with next of kin or guardian and attempt transfer. Criminal liability for falsification, concealment.

Idaho Natural Death Act, Idaho Code secs. 39-4501-4508 (1977).
Written declaration signed in presence of two disinterested witnesses. Prescribed form in statute. Revocation at any time. Effective for five years. Immunity from civil and criminal liability for physician and health facility for compliance.

Indiana Living Wills and Life-Prolonging Act, House Enrolled Act No. 1075, Effective 9/1/85.
Written declaration signed in presence of two disinterested witnesses. Two forms in statute to be substantially followed, but specific additional directions allowed. Living Will form for withholding or withdrawal, Life-Prolonging Procedures form for use of such procedures. Physician to be notified and copy of declaration to be placed in medical record. Living will form considered presumptive evidence of declarant's desires; Life-Prolonging Procedures form obligates physician. Revocation at any time by any method. Immunity for physician, health care provider, or employee for good faith compliance. Unwilling physician to transfer but if unable to do so, must follow specific relocation procedures. Civil and criminal penalties for falsification or concealment.

Iowa Life-Sustaining Procedures Act (1985).
Written declaration signed in presence of two witnesses. Form in statute but modifications allowed. Declarant to give physician copy of declaration. Revocation at any time. Invalid during pregnancy. If no declaration, life-sustaining procedures may be withheld or withdrawn from patient in terminal condition and who is unable to

communicate when specific procedure followed: consultation and written agreement between physician and surrogate as outlined in statute, in presence of witness. Unwilling physician or provider to try to transfer. Immunity for physician, health care provider, or other acting under physician's direction. Criminal penalties for falsification or concealment.

Illinois Living Will Act, Ill. Ann. Stat. ch. 110 ½ secs. 701-710 (Smith-Hurd 1984).

Written declaration executed with same formalities as valid will under Probate Act. Form in statute, but modifications allowed. Invalid during pregnancy. Revocation at any time. Declarant to notify physician, and physician to place copy in medical record. Unwilling physician to transfer patient. Immunity from civil and criminal liability for physician, licensed health care professional, medical care facility or employee thereof for compliance in good faith. Criminal penalties for falsification and concealment.

Kansas Natural Death Act, Kan. Stat. Ann. secs. 65-28, 101-109 (1979).

Written declaration signed in presence of two disinterested witnesses. Form in statute but modifications allowed. Invalid during pregnancy. Revocation at any time. Physician to comply or transfer or be guilty of unprofessional conduct. Immunity from civil or criminal liability for physician, licensed health care professional, medical care facility or employee thereof for compliance. Criminal penalties for falsification and concealment.

Louisiana Life-Sustaining Procedures, La. Rev. Stat. secs. 40:1299.58.1-.10 (1984).

Written declaration signed in presence of two disinterested witnesses. Oral declaration in presence of physician and two witnesses subsequent to terminal diagnosis. Form in statute but modifications allowed. Physician to be notified of declaration and to put it in medical record. If oral, physician to note in record. Revocation at any time. Procedures for decision in absence of declaration, based on agreement between physician and specified surrogate. Procedures for execution of document on behalf of terminally ill minor; certification by court required. Physician to comply with declaration or transfer. Immunity from civil or criminal liability for health care facility, physician or other acting under physician's direction. Criminal penalties for falsification or concealment.

Mississippi Act, Senate Bill No. 2364, ch. 365, Laws of 1984.

Written declaration signed in presence of two disinterested witnesses. Form for declaration in statute but modifications allowed; must be filed with state board of health. Revocation in writing in presence of two disinterested witnesses. Form in statute but modifications allowed; must be filed with state board of health; however, if declarant unable to revoke in writing, may be oral. Physician must report and receive copy of document from board of health before complying. Unwilling physician or medical facility must cooperate in transfer. Immunity for physician for compliance. Criminal penalties for falsification or concealment.

Montana Living Will Act, H.B. 228, Effective 10/1/85.

Written declaration signed in presence of two witnesses. Form provided, but variations allowed. Declarant to notify physician who will make copy part of medical records. Revocation at any time, in any manner. Unwilling physician or facility to make reasonable effort to transfer. Immunity for physician, person under physician's direction, and facility from civil or criminal liability for following declaration. Criminal sanctions for falsification and concealment. Declaration executed in other state in manner substantially similar is effective in Montana.

Nevada Withholding or Withdrawal of Life-Sustaining Procedures, Nev. Rev. Stat. secs. 449.540-690 (1977).

Written declaration executed in same manner as a will, except disinterested witnesses required. Form in statute, but modifications allowed. Physician to give weight to declaration but may consider other factors. Revocation at any time. Immunity for hospital, other health care facility, physician or person working under physician's direction for compliance or failure to comply. Penalties for falsification or concealment.

New Mexico Right to Die Act, N.M. Stat. Ann. secs. 24-7-1-11 (1977).

Document executed with same formalities as required by probate act. Provision of execution on behalf of a minor. Revocation at any time. Immunity for physician, hospital or medical institution or its employees for compliance or failure to comply. Penalties for falsification or concealment.

North Carolina Right to Natural Death Act, N.C. Gen. Stat. secs. 90-320-322 (1977, amend. 1979, 1981, 1983).

Written declaration signed in presence of two disinterested witnesses and proved by certification of a court clerk or notary. Form in statute. Revocation at any time. Immunity for any person, institution or facility for compliance. In absence of declaration, withdrawal or withholding allowed if agreement of spouse, guardian, majority of relatives, or, if none available, attending physician.

Oregon Rights with Respect to Terminal Illness, Or. Rev. Stat. secs. 97.050-.090 (1977, amend. 1983).

Written declaration signed in presence of two disinterested witnesses. If patient in nursing home, one witness must be state-appointed. Form in statute. Revocation at any time. Effective for five years. Physician to note in medical record. Unwilling physician to make effort to transfer. No duty for physician, licensed health professional or medical facility to participate in directive. Immunity for physician, licensed health professional, and health facility for compliance. Penalties for falsification or concealment.

Texas Natural Death Act, Tex. Stat. Ann. Art. 4590h (1977, amend. 1983).

Written declaration signed in presence of two disinterested witnesses. Form in statute. Execution/re-execution after terminal diagnosis. Revocation at any time. Immunity for physician, health facility, health care professional for compliance. Penalties for falsification or concealment.

Vermont Terminal Care Document, Vt. Stat. Ann. tit. 18, secs. 5251-5262 and tit. 13 sec. 1801 (1982).

Written declaration signed in presence of two disinterested witnesses. Form in statute, but modifications allowed. Duty to deliver document to physician or hospital. Revocation at any time. Physician to comply or transfer. Immunity from civil or criminal liability for physician, nurse, health professional, or hospital for compliance. Criminal penalties for falsification or concealment.

Virginia Natural Death Act, Va. Code secs. 54-325.8:1-13 (1983).
Written declaration signed in presence of two witnesses.
Oral declaration in presence of physician and two
witnesses. Physician to be notified and place in record.
Suggested form in statute. Revocation at any time. In
absence of declaration, life-prolonging procedures may be
withdrawn or withheld in appropriate circumstances
when agreement between physician and specified persons. Unwilling physician to transfer. Immunity from civil
or criminal liability for health care facility, physician or
person acting under physician's direction. Criminal
penalties for falsification or concealment.

**Washington Natural Death Act, Wash. Rev. Code Ann. secs.
70.122.010-70.122.905 (1979).**
Written declaration signed in presence of two disinterested witnesses. Form in statute, but modifications
allowed. Physician to place in medical record. Unwilling
physician to make effort to transfer. Revocation at any
time. Immunity for physician, licensed health personnel,
and health facility. Penalties for falsification and
concealment.

**West Virginia Natural Death Act, W.Va. Code, ch. 16, art. 30 secs. 1-10
(1984).**
Written declaration signed in presence of two disinterested witnesses. Form in statute but modifications
allowed. Physician to be notified of declaration and to
place in medical record. All health care facilities to
develop system to identify chart containing declaration.
Revocation at any time. Unwilling physician to transfer
patient. Immunity for physician, licensed health care professional, health facility or employee thereof. Criminal
penalties for falsification and concealment.

**Wisconsin Natural Death Act, Wisc. Stat. secs. 154.01 *et seq.* as
created by 1983 Wisconsin Act 202 (1984).**
Written declaration signed in presence of two disinterested witnesses. Effective for five years. Form in statute.
Revocation at any time. Immunity for physician, inpatient
health care facility, and health care professional acting
under physician's direction. Penalties for falsification and
concealment.

Wyoming Act, Wy. Stat. 33-26 secs. 144-151 (1984).
Written declaration signed in presence of two disinterested witnesses. Declarant to notify physician. Physician to place in medical record. Form in statute but modifications allowed. Revocation at any time. Physician to comply or transfer. Immunity for physician, licensed health care professional, medical care facility or employee thereof. Penalties for falsification and concealment.

Appendix E

Durable Power of Attorney for Health Care

Although all states have durable power of attorney laws, it is uncertain whether this power may be used to make health care decisions which authorize withholding or withdrawal of life-sustaining treatment for the incompetent principal who is in a terminal condition. Only three states have specifically amended their laws to address health care decisions. It is important to consult with an attorney as to other official statements regarding this subject, e.g., attorney general's opinions.

California

Calif. Civil Code 2430-2433 (1983).
Authorizes refusal of life-sustaining treatment on behalf of incompetent principal. Refusal to be based on prestated wishes of principal. Detailed appointment procedures. Immunity to attorney-in-fact and physician for compliance with principal's wishes.

Colorado

Colo. Rev. Stat. sec. 15-14-501 as amended 1983 by L.83, p.661, sec. 1.
As illustration of attorney-in-fact authority, "power to consent to or approve on behalf of principal any medical or other professional care, counsel, treatment or service" by health care professionals or institutions. No specificity regarding termination of treatment.

Pennsylvania

Pa. Cons. Stat. Ann. secs. 5601-5607 (1982).
Authorizes agent to give directions regarding medical care. Specifies only consent, not refusal.

American Hospital Association

Policy

A Patient's Bill of Rights

Patient and Community Relations

This policy document presents the official position of the American Hospital Association as approved by the Board of Trustees and House of Delegates.

The American Hospital Association presents a Patient's Bill of Rights with the expectation that observance of these rights will contribute to more effective patient care and greater satisfaction for the patient, his physician, and the hospital organization. Further, the Association presents these rights in the expectation that they will be supported by the hospital on behalf of its patients, as an integral part of the healing process. It is recognized that a personal relationship between the physician and the patient is essential for the provision of proper medical care. The traditional physician-patient relationship takes on a new dimension when care is rendered within an organizational structure. Legal precedent has established that the institution itself also has a responsibility to the patient. It is in recognition of these factors that these rights are affirmed.

1. The patient has the right to considerate and respectful care.

2. The patient has the right to obtain from his physician complete current information concerning his diagnosis, treatment, and prognosis in terms the patient can be reasonably expected to understand. When it is not medically advisable to give such information to the patient, the information should be made

During the 1970s the American Hospital Association's Board of Trustees had a Committee on Health Care for the Disadvantaged, which developed the *Statement on a Patient's Bill of Rights.* That document was approved by the AHA House of Delegates on February 6, 1973, and has been published in various forms. This reprinting and reclassification conforms with the current classification system for AHA documents. The contents are unchanged.

available to an appropriate person in his behalf. He has the right to know, by name, the physician responsible for coordinating his care.

3. The patient has the right to receive from his physician information necessary to give informed consent prior to the start of any procedure and/or treatment. Except in emergencies, such information for informed consent should include but not necessarily be limited to the specific procedure and/or treatment, the medically significant risks involved, and the probable duration of incapacitation. Where medically significant alternatives for care or treatment exist, or when the patient requests information concerning medical alternatives, the patient has the right to such information. The patient also has the right to know the name of the person responsible for the procedures and/or treatment.

4. The patient has the right to refuse treatment to the extent permitted by law and to be informed of the medical consequences of his action.

5. The patient has the right to every consideration of his privacy concerning his own medical care program. Case discussion, consultation, examination, and treatment are confidential and should be conducted discreetly. Those not directly involved in his care must have the permission of the patient to be present.

6. The patient has the right to expect that all communications and records pertaining to his care should be treated as confidential.

7. The patient has the right to expect that within its capacity a hospital must make reasonable response to the request of a patient for services. The hospital must provide evaluation, service, and/or referral as indicated by the urgency of the case. When medically permissible, a patient may be transferred to another facility only after he has received complete information and explanation concerning the needs for and alternatives to such a transfer. The institution to which the patient is to be transferred must first have accepted the patient for transfer.

8. The patient has the right to obtain information as to any relationship of his hospital to other health care and educational institutions insofar as his care is concerned. The patient has the

right to obtain information as to the existence of any professional relationships among individuals, by name, who are treating him.

9. The patient has the right to be advised if the hospital proposes to engage in or perform human experimentation affecting his care of treatment. The patient has the right to refuse to participate in such research projects.

10. The patient has the right to expect reasonable continuity of care. He has the right to know in advance what appointment times and physicians are available and where. The patient has the right to expect that the hospital will provide a mechanism whereby he is informed by his physician or a delegate of the physician of the patient's continuing health care requirements following discharge.

11. The patient has the right to examine and receive an explanation of his bill regardless of source of payment.

12. The patient has the right to know what hospital rules and regulations apply to his conduct as a patient.

No catalog of rights can guarantee for the patient the kind of treatment he has a right to expect. A hospital has many functions to perform, including the prevention and treatment of disease, the education of both health professionals and patients, and the conduct of clinical research. All these activities must be conducted with an overriding concern for the patient, and above all, the recognition of his dignity as a human being. Success in achieving this recognition assures success in the defense of the rights of the patient.

Appendix G

'Do Not Resuscitate' Guidelines for Hospitals and Physicians *

*Reprinted with permission of the Medical Society of New York State.

The following are intended only to be guidelines for physicians and hospitals. Hospital medical staffs and governing bodies are encouraged to develop policies consistent with their respective bylaws and rules and regulations.

Definition

DNR (Do Not Resuscitate) means that, in the event of a cardiac or respiratory arrest, cardiopulmonary resuscitative measures will not be initiated or carried out.

Background

1. An appropriate knowledge of the serious nature of the patient's medical condition is necessary.

2. The attending physician should determine the appropriateness of a DNR order for any given patient.

3. DNR orders are compatible with maximal therapeutic care. A patient may receive vigorous support in all other therapeutic modalities and yet a DNR order may be justified.

4. When a patient is capable of making his own judgments, the DNR decision should be reached consensually by the patient and physician. When the patient is not capable of making his own decision, the decision should be reached after consultation between the appropriate family member(s) and the physician. If a patient disagrees, or, in the case of a patient incapable of making an appropriate decision, the family member(s) disagree, a DNR order should not be written.

Implementation

1. Once the DNR decision has been made, this directive shall be written as a formal order by the attending physician. A verbal or telephone order for DNR cannot be justified as a sound medical or legal practice.

2. It is the responsibility of the attending physician to insure that this order and its meaning are discussed with appropriate members of the hospital staff.

3. The facts and considerations relevant to this decision shall be recorded by the attending physician in the progress notes.

4. The DNR order shall be subject to review at any time by all concerned parties on a regular basis and may be rescinded at any time.

Council 9/9/82

American Hospital Association

AHA

Guidelines

Discharge Planning

Health Care Delivery

This guideline document is intended to provide general advice to the membership of the American Hospital Association, as approved by the General Council.

Introduction

The American Hospital Association believes that coordinated discharge planning functions are essential for hospitals to maintain high-quality patient care. Discharge planning is important because it facilitates appropriate patient and family decision making. In addition, it can also help reduce length of stay and the rate of increase of health care costs.

For most patients, discharge planning is a part of routine patient care. For those patients whose posthospital needs are expected to be complex, special discharge planning services are warranted. These guidelines present general information for organizing services for complex discharge planning.

It is recognized that each hospital has different resources and organizes its services differently to meet specific patient needs. It is further recognized that rapid changes in the hospital environment cause rapid changes in discharge planning. These changes, however, have emphasized the importance of discharge planning, and it is in that context that these guidelines are presented.

These guidelines were developed by the Society for Hospital Social Work Directors of the American Hospital Association to assist hospitals in evaluating and improving their discharge planning functions. This guidelines document recognizes that each hospital must conduct this function according to its own needs, its resources, and the needs of its patients. It was approved by the General Council on April 11-12, 1984.

Definition

Discharge planning is an interdisciplinary hospitalwide process that should be available to aid patients and their families in developing a feasible posthospital plan of care.

Purposes

The purposes of discharge planning are to ensure the continuity of high-quality patient care, the availability of the hospital's resources for other patients requiring admission, and the appropriate utilization of resources. To ensure the continuity of high-quality care, the hospital will:

• Assign responsibility for the coordination of discharge planning

• Identify as early as possible, sometimes before hospital admission, the expected posthospital care needs of patients utilizing admission and preadmission screening and review programs when available

• Develop with patients and their families appropriate discharge care plans

• Assist patients and their families in planning for the supportive environment necessary to provide the patients' posthospital care

• Develop a plan that considers the medical, social, and financial needs of patients

To ensure the availability of hospital resources for subsequent patients with due regard for prospective pricing, the hospital's procedures should be carried out in such a manner as to accomplish timely discharge.

Principles of Discharge Planning

The discharge planning process incorporates a determination of the patient's posthospital care preferences, needs, the patient's capacity for self-care, an assessment of the patient's living conditions, the identification of health or social care resources needed to assure high-quality posthospital care, and the counseling of the patient or family to prepare them for posthospital care. Discharge planning should be carried out in keeping with varying community resources and hospital utilization activities.

Discharge Planning when Multiple Resources are Required

In addition to discharge instructions for each routine patient discharge plan, the coordination of multiple resources may be required to achieve continued safe and high-quality posthospital care in situations where the patient's needs are complicated.

Essential Elements

The essential elements in accomplishing the hospital's goals for high-quality, cost-effective patient care are:

- *Early Identification of Patients Likely to Need Complex Posthospital Care*

There are certain factors that may indicate a need for early initiation of discharge planning, either before admission or upon admission. Screens for automatic early patient identification are developed for each specialty service by the physician and relevant health care providers and used as guidelines to carry out discharge planning.

- *Patient and Family Education*

With greater emphasis on self-care, patient and family education is critical to successful discharge planning. The coordination of discharge planning must integrate teaching about physical care to facilitate appropriate self-care in the home.

- *Patient/Family Assessment and Counseling*

The psychosocial and physical assessment and counseling of patients and families to determine the full range of needs upon discharge and to prepare them for the posthospital stage of care is a dynamic process. This process includes evaluation of the patient's and the family's strengths and weaknesses; the patient's physical condition; understanding the illness and treatment; the ability to assess the patient's and family's capacities to adapt to changes; and, where necessary, to assist the persons involved to manage in their continued care. Discharge planning and the coordination of posthospital care plans requires an ability to adapt the plans to meet changes in the patient's condition.

• *Plan Development*

The discharge plan development should include the results of the assessment and the self-care instructions, including information from the patient, the family, and all relevant health care professionals. Service needs and options are identified, and the patient and family are helped to understand the consequences of whatever plan they choose to adopt. A supportive climate is critical to facilitate appropriate decision making.

• *Plan Coordination and Implementation*

The hospital achieves high-quality and effective discharge planning through the delegation of specific responsibilities to the principal and specialized disciplines providing care. In order to minimize the potential for fragmented care and to fulfill the need for a central hospital linkage to the community, there should be assigned responsibility for discharge planning coordination for complex cases.

• *Postdischarge Follow-Up*

In complex situations requiring coordinated discharge planning, the plans should ensure follow-up with the patient, the family, and/or community service(s) providing continued care to determine the discharge plan outcome.

• *Quality Assurance*

The quality of the discharge planning system should be monitored through the hospitalwide quality assurance program.

Appendix I

Adjunct Legal Task Force on Biomedical Ethics

Report of the Adjunct Legal Task Force on Biomedical Ethics

The Adjunct Legal Task Force on Biomedical Ethics was formed in 1983 by the Office of Legal and Regulatory Affairs of the American Hospital Association and the American Academy of Hospital Attorneys in order to address legal issues in the complex and rapidly changing area of biomedical ethics. The Task Force prepared this analysis of the legal issues involved in the establishment of institutional ethics committees.

From the American Hospital Association:
Richard L. Epstein, Senior Vice President
Mary Layne Ahern, Staff Attorney, Office of Legal and Regulatory Affairs

From the American Academy of Hospital Attorneys:
George J. Annas, Boston University School of Public Health (Boston, MA)
Stephen M. Blaes, Blaes and Heath (Wichita, KS)
Teresa A. Brooks, Dykema, Gossett, Spencer, Goodnow & Trigg (Detroit, MI)
Alex M. Clarke, Baird, Holm, McEachen, Pedersen, Hamann & Strasheim (Omaha, NE)
William J. Curran, Harvard Medical School (Boston, MA)
Edward B. Goldman, University of Michigan Hospitals (Ann Arbor, MI)
Nina Novak, Miles & Stockbridge (Washington, DC)
Stuart Orsher, M.D. (New York, NY)
J. Stuart Showalter, The Catholic Health Association, Inc. (St. Louis, MO)

Introduction

An institutional ethics committee can be of considerable benefit to a hospital as it struggles with the current complex biomedical ethical environment. Although not a panacea for ethical dilemmas, an ethics committee may provide assurance to patients, the medical staff, the community, and courts that careful, thoughtful, and compassionate decision-making devices exist within a hospital.

Most of the literature on institutional ethics committees contains a paragraph or two on the legal considerations attendant to the establishment and functioning of such committees. These paragraphs generally refer to the confidentiality requirements for medical records, and occasionally to the provision of immunity for committee members. However, the legal aspects of ethics committees are much greater in number and broader in scope than this. It is important that a committee's general purpose includes a discussion of potential issues concerning legal rights or compliance with laws. The committee can use the law to provide it with guidelines in sorting out the often conflicting goals of individuals and society.

This report will begin with a discussion of a hospital's approach to the question of whether an ethics committee may be a useful and desirable mechanism for the particular community or institution. It will then outline the possible functions of a committee, which may be adapted to address identified issues and problems. A discussion of the form and structure of a committee will follow, highlighting the legal issues. The final section will address the various laws that should be considered in order to provide guidance to a committee.

Hospital Approach

There is no legal duty on the part of a hospital to create a biomedical ethics committee. Neither a statutory nor a common law duty exists as yet. The federal government has not mandated the existence of ethics committees in hospitals that receive federal financial assistance, and no state law requires the establishment of such committees. However, the U. S. Department of Health and Human Services (HHS) has encouraged the creation of such committees. The now-invalid final "Baby Doe" rule included model guidelines for the establishment of Infant Care Review Committees.[1] Although this rule has been declared invalid in *American Hospital Association v. Heckler,*[2] the precedent for government encouragement of the committee concept, at least in a variation tailored to situations involving seriously ill newborns, has been set. The Child Abuse Amendments of 1984, which include "Baby Doe" provisions, also include language that gives the Secretary authority to develop model guidelines:

> . . . to encourage the establishment within health-care facilities of committees which would serve the purposes of educating hospital personnel and families of disabled infants with life-threatening conditions, recommending institutional policies and

1) 45 C.F.R. Part 84, Nondiscrimination on the Basis of Handicap; Procedures and Guidelines Relating to Health Care for Handicapped Infants (Jan. 12, 1984).

2) *American Hospital Association v. Heckler,* No. 84-6211 (2d Cir. Dec. 27, 1984), petition for certiorari filed March 27, 1985.

3) Pub. L. 98-457. Final rule implementing statute at 45 C.F.R. Part 1340.15, *Fed. Reg.* Vol. 50, No. 72, pp. 14879-14901 (April 15, 1985).

4) See, e.g., *In re Conservatorship of Rudolfo Torres,* No. C1-84-761, Minn. Sup. Ct. (Nov. 2, 1984); *In re Hamlin,* No. 49101-1, Wash. Sup. Ct. (Nov. 1, 1984); *In re L.H.R.,* No. 41065, Ga. Sup. Ct. (Oct. 16, 1984); *In re Storar,* 420 N.E. 2d 64 (N.Y. 1981), rev'd, *In re Storar,* 443 N.Y.S. 2d 388, aff'd, *Eichner v. Dillon,* 426 N.Y.S.2d 517 (App. Div. 1980); *Superintendent of Belchertown School v. Saikewicz,* 370 N.E.2d 417 (Mass. 1977).

5) *In re Quinlan,* 355 A.2d 647 (N.J. 1976), cert. denied, 427 U.S. 1922 (1976).

6) See, e.g., *In re L.H.R.,* note 4.

guidelines concerning the withholding of medically indicated treatment from such infants, and offering counsel and review in cases involving disabled infants with life-threatening conditions.[3]

No court has indicated that an ethics committee is mandated by any overall legal duty, although an increasing number of decisions have included statements on the subject. Some of these decisions speak favorably of the process of consultation with an ethics committee when there is a difficult case, but others are guarded about such a process.[4] The single instance of an official statement regarding the establishment of ethics committees is the New Jersey Attorney General Opinion, which followed the New Jersey Supreme Court decision in the case of Karen Ann Quinlan. However, this decision, advocating intra-institutional discussion of such cases, basically advocated a committee of physicians for the purpose of confirming prognosis rather than a multidisciplinary committee with a number of different purposes.[5]

In the absence of an affirmative legal duty to create a biomedical ethics committee, hospitals should carefully evaluate the reasons for having such a committee. Although relatively new and untried, ethics committees hold great potential for providing education and guidance, and both the public and the courts appear to be impressed by such careful and thoughtful study.[6] Another reason for establishing a committee may be to provide a forum within the hospital so that it can become the mechanism for bringing together differing views and for mediating the frustrations expressed by all concerned, i.e., patients, families, physicians, and other hospital staff members when dealing with difficult ethical problems.

There may be a myriad of biomedical ethical issues within the hospital that would provide the impetus for development of an ethics committee. Following is a list, by no means exhaustive, of such issues within a hospital:

- DNR orders
- Informed consent
- Patient's right to refuse treatment
- Appropriate withholding or withdrawal of life-support systems
- Implementation of mechanisms valid under Living Will/Natural Death Acts
- Special considerations for infants and minors, and dealing with surrogates

- Advice on implications of new services and technology
- Allocation and use of intensive care unit beds
- Confidentiality/patient privacy and other patients rights issues

A hospital should carefully assess its existing resources, in light of the biomedical ethical issues that demand attention. For example, current hospital structure may include a quality assurance committee, a risk management office, a nursing practices committee, a patient care committee, and medical staff committees that may be looking at one or more of these ethical issues. A patient relations department, attorney's office, and various financial offices that may deal with such issues as scheduling and discharge planning, may be resources on the issues. An ethics committee could provide a central role in the internal coordination of an approach to a particular problem.

Functions

Generally, the objectives of an ethics committee are to provide a forum for discussion of issues and cases, to educate, to prospectively analyze policies and protocols, and to provide advice to and build rapport among medical disciplines.[7] In the current complex medical-technological health care environment, the most important function of an ethics committee may be to educate. By providing educational programs and forums for discussion for the hospital and the community on the importance of integration of medical and ethical issues, the committee can underscore the hospital's commitment to enhancing the knowledge of all concerned about these serious issues. For example, the hard questions surrounding pressure to contain health care costs and resulting allocation of resources will be discussed at the community level, with the understanding that progress to national solutions is the ultimate goal. On the institutional level, staff-oriented programs may be designed to share perspectives on relating ethical principles to specific types of patient cases. When a committee's purposes are to educate and to provide a forum for the airing of differing views, the possibility of alleviating problems or reducing potential liability for the hospital is enhanced.

Another frequently mentioned function for an ethics committee is as a resource for evaluation and recommendation of hospital policies on biomedical ethical issues.

7) See, e.g., American Hospital Association, *Guidelines on Hospital Ethics Committees,* approved 1984 (see p. 35 of *Values in Conflict*); *President's Commission for the Study of Ethical Problems in Medicine and Biomedical and Behavioral Research: Deciding to Forego Life-Sustaining Treatment,* Washington, DC: Government Printing Office, 1983; American Academy of Pediatrics: Guidelines for Infant Bioethics Committees (distributed at a National Press Conference on April 27, 1984, in Washington, DC). Evanston, IL: AAP: 1984.

For example, a committee may formulate a policy on do-not-resuscitate orders that would be presented to the board of trustees for approval. A "cookbook" of policies dealing with specific medical situations should be avoided, e.g., for an infant with a specific diagnosis, as such policies may inappropriately intrude upon medical management of a case. However, committee recommendations can help integrate ethical considerations with medical judgments, and may suggest steps in an approach to appropriate decision making. A cautionary note here: although a committee may be communicating directly with the hospital administration and staff in setting up educational programs and discussion forums, it should be careful to avoid communicating any policy innovation or change directly to the staff absent specific authorization.

The characterization of an ethics committee as a review and consultative body to the decision makers in an individual patient's care, even when it is made clear that the committee has no actual decision-making capacity, must be carefully considered by the board, administration, or other body authorizing the committee. Although the benefits of such a committee's function may be considerable, i.e., assurance to the community and to courts that there is a thoughtful decision-making review mechanism within the hospital, the decision to offer consultation of this type must be made with full cognizance of attendant procedural issues.[8] For example, formality of review and mandatory case reporting may lead to implications of affirmative duties in decision making for both the committee and the medical staff.

Any definition of a committee's function as one of "decision making" should be avoided. The potential legal implications of such a role include conflict with patient autonomy, appearance of the corporate practice of medicine, and the strong possibility of more judicial involvement. There are also questions of greater procedural burdens regarding, for example, access and appeals to the committee. Questions of procedures and structures will be discussed in sections following. In addition, the concept of a "retrospective review" of cases function should be carefully scrutinized. The spectre of after-the-fact fault-finding may be counterproductive to the committee, reducing medical staff cooperation, as well as leading to a "watchdog" approach implying a duty of care on the part of the committee. There are existing committees within

8) See pages 97-99.

the hospital that have responsibility for conducting appropriate reviews.

Form/Structure

Authority. A biomedical ethics committee generally may be structured as a committee of either the medical staff or the governing board. The relative merits of one type of committee over another should be analyzed in light of the functions it is meant to fulfill, attendant legal rights and responsibilities, and, of course, within the context of the size and kind of hospital considering establishment.

A medical staff-authorized committee raises two threshold questions: what kind of control will the hospital have over such a medical staff committee? and what is the level of liability of such a committee? First, a change in bylaws may be required to authorize such a committee. Second, there may be an effect on the independence of an investigation into the facts of a particular case with this type of committee. However, the confidentiality of patient and committee information may be more easily and effectively preserved within this structure.[9] Finally, the physician-dominated medical-staff authorized ethics committee may become a "prognosis" committee with the purpose of confirming prognosis, but without the broad functions of an institutional ethics committee. The medical staff-authorized ethics committee may not be the preferred structure in light of the reasons for establishing a committee, e.g., achieving a broader focus in approaching issues minimizing liability and providing an open forum for independent discussion.

9) See discussion, pp. 93-94.

A hospital committee, i.e., governing board-authorized, may achieve a broader range of desired functions, including education, policy recommendation, and forum for resolution of biomedical ethical issues. For example, a hospital committee can generally reflect a diversity of membership possible with an institutional structure. As such, it may have several benefits in terms of independence and avoidance of bias in its consideration of policies and particular cases, e.g., conflicts of interests on the part of physician members may be minimized. The following section will discuss the implications of such a structure in greater detail. However, it is useful to note that a broad view of an ethics committee's functions to include both community and intra-institutional education and institutional policy-making may generally result in a committee authorized by the governing board rather than the medical staff.

Values in Conflict

Procedural Issues. A biomedical ethics committee should have established, written procedures in order to best achieve its goals. Procedural issues include (1) convening members from a cross-section of the medical staff, hospital governing board and administration, and community; (2) deciding on an appropriate method of meeting on a regular schedule and on response time to issues brought to it; (3) determining who has access to the committee, i.e., who has standing to bring a case to the committee for discussion, and at what times; and (4) establishing a format for meetings and proper methods for handling information both brought to, and released by, the committee.

The procedural issues to be addressed will vary depending upon the functions that the committee will undertake. There may be considerable variation between the procedures for meetings where there is to be consideration of an individual case, and meetings to discuss educational programs or recommendation of policy. For example, different procedures may be desired regarding attendance of members and of "invitees," and methods of taking and recording members' votes when a policy is being recommended versus when a specific patient's case is being discussed.

The problems of keeping committee records and of committee access to patient records are among the most troublesome legal problems confronting an ethics committee. First, the hospital, and the ethics committee by extension, are bound by the customary laws and regulations regarding medical record confidentiality,[10] the length and method of retention of such records,[11] and patient access to his or her own record.[12] In addition, patient or appropriate surrogate consent is required before any confidential patient information may be disclosed to anyone outside of the patient/health care professional relationship. Therefore, an ethics committee with members who are from "outside" the hospital, such as community representatives, may be subject to liability if confidential patient information is used in discussion of a case without patient consent. Also, invitees to a committee meeting, even family members in some cases, may not have access to patient information without consent. In order to circumvent potential problems of this type, a hospital could consider strategies such as extending confidentiality policy to cover nonhospital members of the committee, appointing such members "dollar-a-year" employees who

[10] JCAH, *Accreditation Manual for Hospitals* (1984); See also, CAL. CIV. CODE, sec. 56.10; N.Y. Pub. Health Law, sec. 4165.

[11] Retention requirements vary considerably from state to state. See, e.g., 7 PA. BULL. 3657, Rules and Regulations for the Licensure of General and Special Hospitals in Virginia.

[12] See, e.g., FLA. STAT. ANN., sec. 395.202; ILL. STAT. ANN., ch. 110, sec. 8-2001; MINN. STAT. ANN., sec. 144.335.

would then agree to a standard oath of nondisclosure, or asking for patient consent on admittance. In any case, a committee should use all possible appropriate methods to keep the patient's identity confidential.

The second consideration of an ethics committee affecting a patient's record is the appropriate recordation of an ethics committee recommendation in that record. A committee's protocols should include how such a recommendation is made and how it is to be recorded, i.e., quorum, voting, and dissent. Hospital policy should be clear as to who will make such an addition, i.e., physician, committee chairman. It should be noted again here that if a committee chooses not to undertake the advisory function, it will not find it necessary to deal with problems of confidentiality regarding a specific patient.

The records or minutes of ethics committee meetings raise questions as to whether such records have any protection from discoverability, and whether they should be open to the public or held in confidence.[13] These are both legal and public policy questions. If confidential patient information is not discussed in committee, then the problem of discoverability fades and the public policy favoring an open process of exchanging information on biomedical ethics rises. If patient information is used in committee discussions, any minutes or case notes should be recorded in such a way as to guarantee patient anonymity.

Immunity of the hospital from liability for committee actions, and of committee members for their actions, is a frequently discussed legal concern. Generally, there are state statutes that provide immunity from civil liability for medical review committee members, and in some states for board of trustee members.[14] These vary considerably from state to state, but generally protect persons involved in committees that evaluate quality of care. An ethics committee may not be protected under such statutes and even read in the best possible light they could provide false security. However, hospitals may wish to propose enactment of a statute specifically immunizing committee members from civil liability, or to structure their insurance appropriately, in the remote possibility that there will be danger to them in establishing ethics committees.

Another important procedural issue is the limit of an ethics committee's jurisdiction. Areas that will not be considered by such a committee should be clearly stated. For example, it may be appropriate to exclude problems of im-

13) State laws dealing with discoverability and admissibility of committee records vary, but generally focus on protection for committees such as medical staff and peer review committees. See, e.g., MICH. STAT. ANN., secs. 14.15 and 14.57; WASH. REV. CODE, sec. 4.24.250.

14) See, e.g., ARIZ. REV. STAT. ANN., sec. 36-445.02; VA. CODE, sec. 8.01-581.16.

Values in Conflict

paired physicians, technology assessment, and institutional review board[15] issues from the committee's topics of concern, since these issues are ordinarily dealt with in other committees. In any case, there should be attention given to proper coordination between an ethics committee and other hospital mechanisms in order to facilitate cooperation and to avoid potentially confusing overlap of responsibilities.

Finally, the role of the attorney must be appropriately structured. A hospital may decide that the attorney who represents the hospital should act as a member of the committee in order to provide legal perspective to committee deliberations when necessary; however, care should be taken to avoid any possible conflict of interest inherent in this arrangement. Another view is that it may be difficult for an attorney to both advise the committee and act as a member. This view would then prompt a structure with an attorney member of the committee chosen from the community, and the hospital's attorney as counsel. It may be unwise for the committee to have its own attorney since it may appear that the committee is not representative of the hospital.

Legal Guidance to an Ethics Committee

There are three broad categories of laws and legal concerns that may aid an ethics committee in fulfillment of the purposes determined for it by the hospital. These categories include societal and legal concerns, prescriptive laws on the state level, and general laws and legal rights best described as those providing guidance on a specific patient's rights. Each of the concerns in these categories will appear in varying degrees of importance when an ethics committee fulfills any of its chosen functions, be it education, policy recommendation, or advisory. However, it is the policy-recommendation function that probably will benefit the most from the examination that follows.

Societal Concerns. The impact of societal concerns on the ethics committee of a hospital may not have been considered when forming the committee. However, they provide an important framework for reference for a committee with a broad mandate, especially in the structuring of hospital policies and educational programs.

Medicare and Medicaid are, of course, the clearest examples of society's decision to provide access to care to significant portions of the population. As articulated by

16) Social Security Act (SSA), sec. 1886(c).

17) E.g., MD. [Health] CODE ANN., sec. 19-201 *et seq.;* MASS. GEN. LAWS ANN., ch. 6A, sec. 31 *et seq.;* N.J. REV. STAT., sec. 262H-4.1 *et seq.;* N.Y. [Pub. Health] LAW, sec. 2803 *et seq.*

18) Pub. L. 98-507.

19) E.g., Illinois Experimental Organ Transplant Act (1984).

20) E.g., Rehabilitation Act of 1973 sec. 504, as amended 29 U.S.C. Sec 794.

government, the programs obviously exert a profound influence over the health of the beneficiaries and over the financial health of the care providers. Various cost containment strategies practiced by the Health Care Financing Administration in the form of the prospective payment system[16] and by certain state governments in the form of rate regulation programs[17] will certainly continue to affect basic issues of access to adequate health care services. In addition, special programs, such as the federally funded Hill-Burton program targeted to the provision of care to medically indigent patients, whether sponsored by government on the federal, state, or local level or by hospitals alone, are expressions of societal concerns about access to care that an ethics committee should consider.

Another of these societal level concerns is organ transplantation, which can be approached as an example of concern over allocation of resources. Although there is currently no federal law that attempts to systemize the allocation of transplants, the Organ Transplant Act[18] passed in 1984 mandates national-level study on the issue; in addition, some states have addressed the issue.[19] However, there are currently questions as to the kinds and costs of transplants the government or other payers will cover. The questions on the "macro" level involve the appropriate use of hospital resources, e.g., allocation for the benefit of a few specific needy patients, for the benefit of the larger community population in the form of funds for the emergency room, or for the society's benefit in research and development. On the "micro" level, the question of allocation may include which patient will receive an available organ and who will make the decision.

A third example of societal concerns focuses on protection from discrimination on the basis of age, race, sex, or handicap.[20] A hospital may wish to empower its ethics committee to consider whether the hospital needs any special policies in order to protect the civil rights of patients and the community it serves.

Prescriptive Laws. State laws that define hospital conduct with respect to certain important protections of specified portions of the community are the prescriptive concerns that an ethics committee should note. For example, states have laws defining minority, which may vary considerably as to the ages covered and the definition of who may be

21) See, e.g., ALA. CODE, sec. 26-1-1, 22-8-4; COLO. REV. STAT., Secs. 13-22-101, 103, 105; OHIO REV. CODE ANN. sec. 3109; VA. CODE, sec. 1-13.42, 54-325.2.

22) Federal regulations implementing the Child Abuse Prevention and Treatment Act of 1973 acknowledge parental rights to choices based on religious beliefs. 45 C.F.R. 1340-1-2(b)(1981).

23) See, e.g., CAL. PEN. CODE, sec. 11161.8, 11165; MISS. CODE ANN. sec. 43-21-351; WISC. STAT. ANN. sec. 48.981.

24) ARIZ. REV. STAT., secs. 36-2281, 2282, 2283 (1984); ILL. ANN. STAT., ch. 23, sec. 2057.1 (1984); LA. REV. STAT. ANN., sec. 40:1299.36 (1984).

25) See note 3.

26) FLA. STAT. ch. 415 (1983). Also see, e.g., N.J.S.A. 52:27G-1 et seq. (defining abuse of elderly as including "willful deprivation of services which are necessary to maintain a person's physical and mental health").

considered a "mature" or "emancipated" minor.[21] Of course, the definitions are crucial as to who may be considered competent for the purpose of giving a valid consent to treatment. An ethics committee may wish to consider educational programs or policies that deal with situations where a minor's consent is questioned. Note that this is an area where sensitive parental rights and rights of religious freedom may come into play.[22]

Extremely important prescriptive state laws are those concerning child abuse and neglect prevention and treatment.[23] Although existing hospital procedures to ensure reporting of cases of suspected abuse or neglect may be adequate, education on the issue may be an appropriate endeavor for the ethics committee.

A few states currently have statutes that specifically focus on problems with treatment decisions for handicapped infants.[24] The federal Child Abuse Amendments of 1984 require state child protective agency regulations to expand the definition of medical neglect, adding the withholding of medically indicated treatment as a prohibited element.[25] An ethics committee may wish to formulate special policies to deal with treatment decisions for handicapped infants, and to arrange educational programs on the issue for its community and state child protective service workers.

Finally, a hospital ethics committee should note that there are certain states that have enacted laws to protect specified groups of adults from abuse and neglect. Generally, these laws focus on the elderly, mentally handicapped, or physically disabled adult and on spousal abuse. A Florida statute, for example, establishes a reporting requirement for physicians, nurses, and other hospital personnel when abuse or neglect of these persons is suspected.[26] The definition of what constitutes "neglect" and whether the definition includes medical neglect are examples of issues that concern a hospital, and an ethics committee may aid in the achievement of smooth compliance with such laws through education programs for the staff and the community.

Guidance. In this category, laws and legal rights should be considered for their impact upon ethics committee functions as they relate to a patient's exercise of his or her rights. The concern here is the proper implementation of an expression of desire to exercise rights. These differ from the laws described in the "Prescriptive" section, which, in and of themselves, mandate conduct. There are two groups of legal concerns in this area: one including broad patient rights and the other addressing a patient's right to choose and refuse treatment.

The first group of legal concerns in this category focuses on basic patient rights, including Patient's Bill of Rights and informed consent. It is not necessary to go into these concerns in detail here, but to point out an ethics committee's connection with the protection of these rights. The American Hospital Association published a statement in 1975 titled "A Patient's Bill of Rights," which has been widely quoted and debated.[27] It contains affirmations of basic rights to care, privacy, confidentiality of information, access to information, and to consent to or refusal of treatment. Certain states have codified variations upon this Bill of Rights, which require hospitals to develop policies describing patients' rights and to provide appropriate notice of such a policy.[28] Whether codified or not, it is an appropriate undertaking for an ethics committee to suggest such a document to the policymaking board of the hospital. Informed consent, although primarily the responsibility of the physician, may deserve special consideration by an ethics committee, which may wish to propose procedures to facilitate the process of informed consent to treatment.[29]

The second group of issues focuses on a patient's right to refuse treatment. For example, the establishment of a do-not-resuscitate order policy in a hospital can be aided by an ethics committee, which can ensure that discussion takes place among the staff on the issue and that educational resources be made available to patients, staff, and family.[30] An ethics committee may similarly be a facilitator in the smooth acceptance of a patient's desires expressed in a Living Will,[31] or under the aegis of a state Natural Death Act[32] or Durable Power of Attorney Act[33] if one exists. Probably the most important function a committee can undertake in these instances is to provide a forum for discussion in the event that one of these methods of prior expression of a patient is controversial or misunderstood. In this way, exacerbation of a problem situation can be avoided.

27) American Hospital Association, Statement, Patient's Bill of Rights (1975) (see appendix B, *Values in Conflict*).

28) See, e.g., MINN. STAT. ANN. sec. 144.651 (West Supp. 1979).

29) See, e.g., Model Health Care Consent Act, Nat'l Conf. of Commissioners on Unif. State Laws (1982).

30) For example, see the DNR guidelines published by the New York State Medical Society.

31) See, e.g., GA. CODE ANN. sec. 31-32-1-12 (1984); ILL. ANN. STAT. ch. 110½ sec. 701-710 (Smith-Hurd 1984).

32) See, e.g., CAL. HEALTH & SAFETY CODE, sec. 7185-7195 (1976); N.M. STAT. ANN. sec. 24-7-1-11 (1977); VA. CODE, sec. 54-325.8 (1983).

33) CAL. CIV. CODE
2430-2433 (1983); COLO.
REV. STAT., sec. 15-14-501
as amended 1983 by L.
83, p. 661, sec. 1; PA.
CONS. STAT. ANN. sec.
5601-5607 (1982).

Conclusion

As a hospital considers methods of integrating a thought-ful approach to biomedical ethical issues into its internal structure and community relationships, it may focus on an institutional ethics committee as an appropriate con-duit to its goals. Although existing committees may be performing some of the functions discussed in this paper, a hospital may wish to centralize the activities in a com-mittee that would help provide education and policy guidelines and be available for consultation. Such a com-mittee could provide support to patients, family, and staff. It could also heighten society's view of the hospital as a conduit to responsible decision making, and be seen as a plus by courts and legislative systems.[33]

Glossary

Biomedical   Associated with the practice of medicine.

Competency   According to law, sufficient mental ability to understand the nature and consequences of one's actions and to make a rational decision.

Death   Has occurred when an individual has sustained either: (1) irreversible cessation of circulatory and respiratory functions, or (2) irreversible cessation of all functions of the entire brain, including the brain stem.

Decision-making capacity   The ability to make choices that reflect an understanding and appreciation of the nature and consequences of one's actions.

DNR (do not resuscitate)   An order that directs that cardiopulmonary resuscitation (CPR) not be initiated.

Durable power of attorney   A written statement appointing another as agent and conferring authority to perform certain specified acts or kinds of acts on the principal's behalf; it remains valid if the principal becomes incompetent. (See Appendix D.)

Ethics   The study of rational processes for determining the most morally desirable course of action in the face of conflicting value choices.

Ethics committee   Usually a hospital committee that may direct educational programs on biomedical ethical issues, provide forums for discussion among hospital and medical professionals and others about biomedical ethical issues, serve in an advisory capacity and/or as a resource to persons involved in biomedical decision making, and evaluate institutional experiences related to review decisions having biomedical ethical implications.

Health care professional

An individual who has received special training or education in a health-related field and/or is licensed or certified in a health-related field. Health professionals include individuals in administration, direct provision of patient care, and support or ancillary services in the hospital.

Informed consent

A process for active and shared decision making between practitioner and patient that involves adequate disclosure (informed) and the element of choice (consent).

Life support system

Refers to respirators, renal dialysis machines, and other equipment that artificially maintains bodily functions.

Living will

Documents by which individuals can indicate their preferences not to be given "heroic" or "extraordinary" treatments. (See Appendix C.)

Mature minor

Person who would normally be a minor under state law but is considered a competent adult according to special state law provisions.

Medical error

An avoidable mistake made in the provision of health care services.

Morals

Particular actions, beliefs, attitudes, and codes of rules concerning concepts of right and proper conduct that characterize different societies, groups, and individuals.

Natural death act

State legislation that protects a patient's directive to a physician. It also spells out in various ways penalties for failing to act in accord with a properly executed directive of a patient. (See Appendix C.)

Negative medical outcome

An unwanted and undesirable effect or side effect of treatment.

Noncompliant patient

An individual who seeks or needs care but fails to follow health care recommendations.

Patient care team

All physicians and other health care professionals involved in the treatment of a particular patient.

Surrogate

Typically a close relative or friend who is named when the patient lacks the capacity to make particular medical decisions.

Values in Conflict

Treatment
A course of therapy and/or medication prescribed by a physician or other qualified health care professional. Medical and legal opinion is not firm as to whether food and water is considered treatment.

Value
Something intrinsically valuable or desirable.

Selected Readings and Resources in Biomedical Ethics

The following bibliography lists only a few of the resources currently available that are germane to the issues highlighted in this report of the Special Committee on Biomedical Ethics; however, readers are encouraged to check their own local resources for additional references. The special committee is especially indebted to the Center for Bioethics Library of The Joseph and Rose Kennedy Institute of Ethics, Georgetown University, Washington, DC, and to its librarians for their assistance in compiling the listing which follows.

General and Reference Documents

American College of Physicians ethics manual. *Annals of Internal Medicine.* 101:129-137, 263-274, 1984.

BIOETHICS (Online Data Base). Available through MEDLARS computer systems of National Library of Medicine. Produced by Kennedy Institute of Ethics, Georgetown University, Washington, DC.

Encyclopedia of Bioethics. Reich, W., editor. New York City: The Free Press, 1978.

Handbook of the Society for the Right To Die (annual listing of living will laws). New York City: Society for the Right To Die.

The Hastings Center Bibliography of Ethics, Biomedicine, and Professional Responsibility. Frederick, MD: University Publications of America, 1984.

Selected reports of the President's Commission for the Study of Ethical Problems in Medicine and Biomedical and Behavioral Research: *Deciding to Forego Life-Sustaining Treatment; Defining Death;* and *Making Health Care Decisions.* Washington, DC: U.S. Government Printing Office, 1981-1983.

Abrams, Natalie, and Buckner, Michael D., editors. *Medical Ethics; A Clinical Textbook and Reference for the Health Care Professions,* The MIT Press, Cambridge, 1983.

Gorovitz, Samuel; Macklin, Ruth; Jameton, Andrew L., and others, editors. *Moral Problems in Medicine.* Englewood Cliffs, NJ: Prentice-Hall, Inc., 1983. Second edition.

Jonsen, Albert R.; Siegler, Mark; and Winslade, William J. *Clinical Ethics.* New York: Macmillan Publishing Co., 1982.

Levine, Carol. *Taking Sides: Clashing Views on Controversial Bio-Ethical Issues.* Guilford, CT: The Dushkin Publishing Group, 1984.

Walters, LeRoy, ed. *Bibliography of Bioethics.* New York City: Macmillan Publishing Co., 1975-. Annual.

Case Studies

Benjamin, Martin, and Curtis, Jay. *Ethics in Nursing.* Oxford University Press, New York City, 1981.

Brody, Howard. *Ethical Decisions in Medicine.* Boston: Little, Brown, 1981.

Levine, Carol; and Veatch, Robert M. *Cases in Bioethics from the Hastings Center Report.* Hastings-on-Hudson, New York City: The Hastings Center, 1983.

Veatch, Robert M. *Case Studies in Medical Ethics.* Cambridge, MA: Harvard University Press, 1977.

Walton, Douglas N. *Ethics of Withdrawal of Life-Support Systems: Case Studies on Decision Making in Intensive Care.* Westport, CT: Greenwood Press, 1983.

Periodicals

Hastings Center Report. Hastings-on-Hudson, New York City: Institute of Society, Ethics, and the Life Sciences.

Ethics Committee Newsletter. Boston: American Society of Law and Medicine.

Organizational Ethics Newsletter. Berkeley, CA: Marvin Brown.

Hospital Ethics. Chicago: American Hospital Association

Audiovisual References

Code Grey: Ethical Dilemmas in Nursing. Achtenberg, Ben, and Sawyer, Joan, in collaboration with Mitchell, Christine; Fanlight Productions, 47 Halifax St., Boston, MA, 1983.

Human Values in Medicine and Health Care: Audio-Visual Resources. Shmavonian, Nadya, compiler. New Haven, CT: Yale University Press, 1983.

Medical Ethics Film Review Project. Hollander, Rachelle, editor. College Park: Council for Philosophical Studies, University of Maryland, 1975.

Books and Articles

Confidentiality

Bok, Sissela. The limits of confidentiality. *The Hastings Center Report* 13(1): 24-31, February 1983.

Journal of the American Medical Association. Confidentiality expectations of patients, physicians, and medical students. *JAMA* 247(19): 2695-2697, May 21, 1982.

Rand Corporation. Federal and state regulations concerning the privacy of health care data. Santa Monica, CA: Rand Paper Series, No. P-5783.

Schuchman, Herman; Foster, Leila; Nye, Sandra, and others. *Confidentiality of Health Records.* New York: Gardner Press, Inc., 1982.

Siegler, Mark. Confidentiality in medicine—a decrepit concept. *New England Journal of Medicine* 307(24): 1518-1521, December 9, 1982.

Wesbury, Stuart A., and Flory, J. Medical confidentiality: can it still be protected? *Health Matrix* 2(2): 79-80, Summer 1984.

Decision-Making

Momeyer, Richard W. Medical decisions concerning non-competent patients. *Theoretical Medicine* 4(3): 275-290, October 1983.

O'Neil, Richard. Determining proxy consent. *Journal of Medicine and Philosophy* 8(4): 389-403, November 1983.

President's Commission for the Study of Ethical Problems in Medicine and Biomedical and Behavioral Research. *Making Health Care Decisions: The Ethical and Legal Implications of Informed Consent in the Patient-Practitioner Relationship.* Washington, DC: U.S. Government Printing Office, 1982.

Siegler, Mark. Decision-making strategy for clinical-ethical problems in medicine. *Archives of Internal Medicine* 142:2178-9, 1982.

Steinbrook, R. and Lo, B. Decision Making for Incompetent Patients by Designated Proxy—California's New Law. *New England Journal of Medicine* 310:1598-1601, 1984.

Disclosure

Ingelfinger, Franz I. Arrogance. *New England Journal of Medicine* 303(26): 1507-1511, December 25, 1980.

Moutsopoulos, Labrini. Truth-telling to patients. *Medicine and Law* 3(3): 237-251, 1984.

Sheldon, M. Truth-telling in medicine. *Journal of the American Medical Association* 247(5): 651-4, February 5, 1982.

Dying Patients

Beauchamp, Tom L., and Perlin, Seymour, editors. *Ethical Issues in Death and Dying.* Englewood Cliffs, NJ: Prentice-Hall, 1978.

Boyles, Michael, and High, Callas M., editors. *Medical Treatment of the Dying: Moral Issues.* Cambridge, MA: Schenkman Publishing Co., 1978.

Doudera, Edward A., and Peters, Douglas J., editors. *Legal and Ethical Aspects of Treating Critically and Terminally Ill Patients.* Ann Arbor, MI: AUPHA Press, 1982.

Wong, Cynthia B., and Swazey, Judith P., editors. *Dilemma of Dying: Policies and Procedures for Decisions Not To Treat.* Boston: G.K. Hall, 1981.

Do-Not-Resuscitate Orders

Brooks, Teresa A. Withholding treatment and orders not to resuscitate. Pages 105-113 in Doudera, A. Edward, and Peters, J. Douglas, editors, *Legal and Ethical Aspects of Treating Critically and Terminally Ill Patients.* Ann Arbor, MI: AUPHA Press, 1982.

Committee on Policy for DNR Decisions, Yale-New Haven Hospital. Report on do not resuscitate decisions. *Connecticut Medicine* 47(8): 477-483, August 1983.

Lee, Melinda A., and Cassel, Christine K. The ethical and legal framework for the decision not to resuscitate. *Western Journal of Medicine* 140(1): 117-121, January 1984.

McPhail, Aileen; Moore, Sean; O'Connor, John, and others. One hospital's experience with a do not resuscitate policy. *Canadian Medical Association Journal* 125(8): 830-836, October 15, 1981.

Read, William Allan. *Hospital's Role in Resuscitation Decisions.* Chicago: The Hospital Research and Educational Trust, 1983.

Wong, Cynthia B., and Swazey, Judith P., editors. Do not resuscitate decisions and their implementation. In *Dilemmas of Dying: Policies and Procedures for Decisions Not To Treat.* Boston: G.K. Hall, 1981.

Education

Bayley, Corrine. Clinical setting enhances bioethics education. *Hospital Progress* 64(12): 30-53, December 1983.

Callahan, Daniel, and others. Ethics tests for medical boards: the state of the question. *Hastings Center Report* 13(3): 20-33, June 1983.

Johnson, Alan G. Teaching medical ethics as a practical subject: observations from experiences. *Journal of Medical Ethics* 9(1): 5-7, March 1983.

Levine, Melvin D.; Scott, Lee; and Curran, William J. Ethics rounds in a children's medical center: evaluation of a hospital-based program for continuing education in medical ethics. *Pediatrics* 60(2): 202-208, August 1977.

Nora, Paul F. Ethics in housestaff training. *American College of Surgeons Bulletin* 69(5): 3-5, May 1984.

Siegler, Mark. A legacy of Osler: teaching clinical ethics at the bedside. *Journal of the American Medical Association* 239(10): 951-956, 6 March 1978.

Ethics Committees

Cranford, Ronald E., and Doudera, A. Edward, editors, *Institutional Ethics Committees and Health Care Decision Making.* Ann Arbor, MI: Health Administration Press, 1984.

Freedman, Benjamin. One philosopher's experience on an ethics committee. *Hastings Center Report* 11(2): 20-22, April 1981.

Kelley, Sr. Margaret John, and McCarthy, Rev. Donald G., editors. *Ethics Committees: A Challenge for Catholic Health Care.* St. Louis, MO: The Catholic Health Association of the United States, 1984.

Levine, Carol. Hospital ethics committees: a guarded prognosis. *Hastings Center Report* 7(3): 25-27, June 1977.

McCormick, Richard A. Ethics committees: promise or peril? *Law, Medicine, and Health Care* 12(4): 150-155, September 1984.

Murphy, Catherine P. The Changing Role of Nurses in Making Ethical Decisions. *Law, Medicine, and Health Care,* 173-175, Sept. 1984.

Randal, Judith. Are ethics committees alive and well? *Hastings Center Report* 13(6): 10-12, December 1983.

Veatch, Robert M. Hospital ethics committees: is there a role? *Hastings Center Report* 7(3): 22-25, June 1977.

Informed Consent

Baron, Charles H. Medicine and human rights: emerging substantive standards and procedural protections for medical decision making within the American family. *Family Law Quarterly* XVII(1): Spring 1983.

Borak, Jonathan, and Veilleux, Suzanne. Informed consent in emergency settings. *Connecticut Medicine* 48(4): 235-239, April 1984.

Connery, John R. Patients' informed consent requires understanding of treatment risks. *Hospital Progress* 65(5): 38-40, May 1984.

Kapp, Marshall B. Adult protective services: convincing the patient to consent. *Law, Medicine, and Health Care* 2(4): 163-167, September 1983.

Rozovsky, Fay A. *Consent to Treatment: A Practical Guide.* Boston: Little, Brown, 1984.

Law and Government

Abram, Morris B., and Wolf, Susan M. Public involvement in medical ethics; a model for government action. *New England Journal of Medicine* 310(1): 627-632, 8 March 1984.

Shelp, Earl E., editor. *Justice and Health Care.* Hingham, MA: Kluwer Boston, Inc., 1981.

Valentine, Steven R. When the law calls life wrong. *Human Life Review* 8(3): 46-54, Summer 1982.

Minors

Gaylin, Willard, and Macklin, Ruth, editors. *Who Speaks for the Child; the Problems of Proxy Consent.* New York: Plenum Press, 1982.

Holder, Angela Roddey. *Legal Issues in Pediatric and Adolescent Medicine.* New York City: John Wiley, 1977.

Melton, Gary B., Koocher, Gerald P., and Saks, Michael J., editors. *Children's Competence To Consent.* New York: Plenum, 1983.

Moore, Randolph Scott, and Hofmann, Adele D., editors. *American Academy of Pediatrics Conference on Consent and Confidentiality in Adolescent Health Care.* Evanston, Illinois: American Academy of Pediatrics, 1982.

The Rights of Teenagers as Patients. New York City: Public Affairs Committee (pamphlet No. 480), 1975.

Moral Convictions

Fenner, Kathleen M. *Ethics and Law in Nursing.* New York: Van Nostrand Reinhold Co., 1980.

Horsley, Jack E. When you can safely refuse an assignment. *RN* 43(2): 93-94 + , February 1980.

Katz, Jay. Why doctors don't disclose uncertainty. *Report of the Hastings Center* 14(1): 35-44, February 1984.

McCarthy, Donald G., and Moraczewski, Albert S., editors. *Moral Responsibility in Prolonging Life Decisions.* St. Louis, MO: Pope John Center, 1981.

Mitchell, Christine. Integrity in inter-professional relationships. Agich, George J., editor. *Responsibility in Health Care;* Boston, Dordrecht, Holland, D. Reidel Publishing Co. 1982. p. 163-184.

Thomasma, David C. Hospitals' ethical responsibilities as technology, regulation grow. *Hospital Progress* 63(12): 74-79, December 1982.

Rationing

Aaron, Henry J., and Schwartz, William B. *The Painful Prescription: Rationing Hospital Care.* Washington, DC: The Brookings Institution, 1984.

Avorn, J. Benefit and Cost Analysis in Geriatric Care. *New England Journal of Medicine* 310: 1294-1301, 1984.

Evans, R.W. Health Care Technology and the Inevitability of Resource Allocation and Rationing Decisions. *Journal of the American Medical Association* 249: 2047-2053, 2208-2219, 1983.

Iglehart, John K. Transplantation: the problem of limited resources. *New England Journal of Medicine* 309(2): 123-8, 14 July 1983.

Johnson, D.E. Life, Death and the Dollar Sign, Medical Ethics and Cost Containment. *Journal of the American Medical Association* 252: 223-224, 1984.

Winslow, Gerald R. *Triage and Justice: The Ethics of Rationing Life-Saving Medical Resources.* Berkeley: University of California Press, 1982.

Refusal of Treatment

Robertson, John A. *The Rights of the Critically Ill* (revised ACLU Guide to the Rights of the Critically Ill and Dying Patients). New York City: Bantam Books, 1983.

Bobrow, Robert. The choice to die. *Psychology Today* 17(6): 70-72, June 1983.

Jackson, D.L., and Youngner, S. Patient autonomy and "death with dignity": some clinical caveats. *New England Journal of Medicine* 301(8): 404-8, August 23, 1979.

Technology and Transplants

Fox, Renee C., and Swazey, Judith P. *The Courage To Fail: A Social View of Organ Transplants and Dialysis.* Chicago: University of Chicago Press, 1978.

Hearing Report on H.R.4080, The National Organ Transplant Act. Subcommittee on Health and the Environment, House Committee on Energy and Commerce. 98th Congress; hearings July 29, October 17, and October 31, 1983. Washington, DC: U.S. Government Printing Office.

Katz, Jay, and Capron, Alexander Morgan. *Catastrophic Diseases: Who Decides What?: A Psychological and Legal Analysis of the Problems of Hemodialysis and Organ Transplantation.* New York City: Russell Sage Foundation, 1975.

Mamana, John P. Ethics and technology: crossroads in decision making. *Trustee* 35(1): 33-38, January 1982.

Simmons, Roberta G.; Klein, Susan D.; and Simmons, Richard L. *Gift of Life: The Social and Psychological Impact of Organ Transplantation.* New York City: John Wiley, 1977.

Terminally Ill Patients

Bayer, R. et al The Care of the Terminally Ill: Morality and Economics. *New England Journal of Medicine* 309:1490-1494, 1983.

Doudera, Edward A., and Peters, J. Douglas, editors. *Legal and Ethical Aspects of Terminally Ill Patients.* Ann Arbor, MI: AUPHA Press, 1982.

Lynn, Joanne, and Childress, James. Must Patients Always be Given Food and Water. *The Hastings Center Report,* 17-21, 13 (5) October 1983.

Massachusetts General Hospital Clinical Care Committee. Optimum care for hopelessly ill patients. *New England Journal of Medicine* 295(7): 362-364, August 12, 1976.

President's Commission for the Study of Ethical Problems in Medicine and Biomedical and Behavioral Research. *Defining Death.* Washington, DC: U.S. Government Printing Office, 1981.

Index

Access, 4, 34-40,41-42,43.44

Administration/administrator/executive management, 4, 5, 20, 30, 34, 39, 42

Advance directives, 4, 12, 20

Aged patients, 3, 11, 27, 28, 43

American Hospital Association, 1, 4

Business leaders, 39

Case studies 3, Appendix B

Chaplains/clergy, 2, 9, 10, 19, 30, 34, 39

Coalitions, 39

Collaborative decision making, 7, 14-15, 20

Communication with patients, 7-9, 14-15, 19, 20, 23-24, 28-29

Community needs, 1, 27, 41, 42

Community representatives, 31, 34

Competency, 9, 10, 11, 103

Confidentiality/privacy, 3, 4, 23-25, 31-32, 35

Continuity of care, 23, 27-28

Continuum of care, 27-28

Courts, 3, 11, 13, 19

Cover-ups, 29

Decision-making capacity, 9-13, 16-17, 103

Dialysis, 41

Discharge planning, 28, Appendix H

Disclosure, 24, 28-30

Do not resuscitate (DNR), 4, 19-21, Appendix G, 103

Durable power of attorney, 4, 12, 13, 17, 59, Appendix E, 103

Education, 2, 4, 8, 10, 24, 26, 28, 32, 34

Educators, 39

Employees, 3, 23, 29, 35

Environment/atmosphere, 2, 23, 24, 28, 29

Errors in care, 23, 28-29, 104

Ethics committee, 4, 10, 19, 21, 28, 30-35, 103

Family, 2, 8, 9, 10, 11, 12, 13, 17, 19, 20, 21, 23, 28, 30, 32, 33, 35

Forgoing life-sustaining treatment, 19-20

Friends, 8, 11, 12, 13, 16, 19, 20

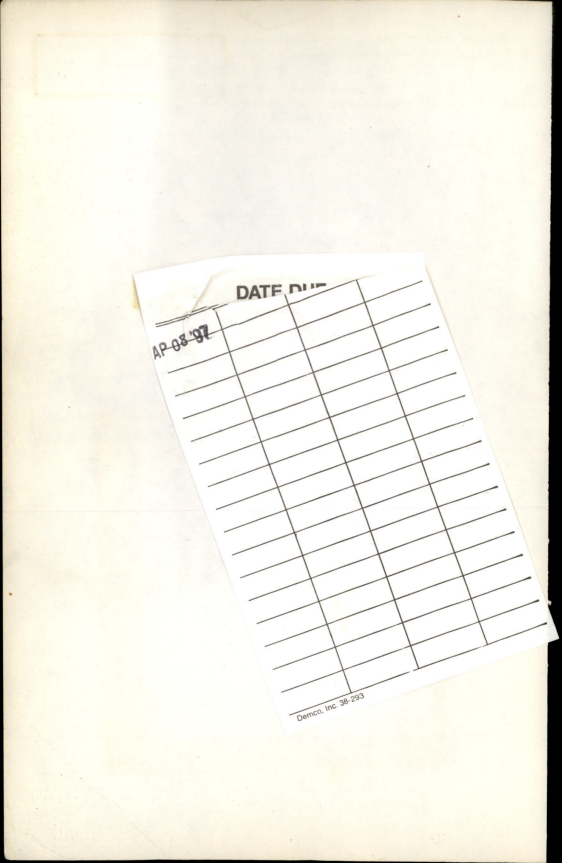